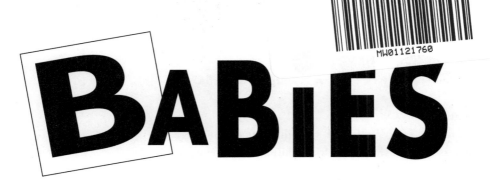

BABIES

FROM TOP
TO BOTTOM

Dr Howard Chilton

Illustrations by Phil Somerville

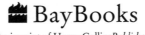 BayBooks

An imprint of HarperCollins*Publishers*

This book is dedicated to my girls, Tamara, Georgina, Isabella.

Acknowledgements
My thanks to Professor Jack Wolfsdorf, who introduced me to
neonatology. Professor Jagdish Gupta, for his always wise counsel.

A Bay Books Publication

Bay Books, an imprint of
HarperCollins*Publishers*
25 Ryde Road, Pymble NSW 2073, Australia
31 View Road, Glenfield, Auckland 10, New Zealand

Revised edition first published by Bay Books in 1994

First edition published by J.B. Fairfax Press in 1990
under the title *The New Baby Book*.

Text Copyright © Howard William Chilton, 1994

National Library of Australia
Cataloguing-in-Publication data:
Chilton, Howard.
    Babies from top to bottom.
    ISBN 1 86378 108 0.

    1. Infants (Newborn) - Care. 2. Infants - Newborn - Nutrition.
    3. Infants - (Newborn) - Health and hygiene. I. Title.
649.122

Cover and internal illustrations by Phillip Somerville.

Printed in Singapore.

9 8 7 6 5 4 3 2 1
97 96 95 94

CONTENTS

About the author

Howard Chilton was born in York, UK, and was breast-fed. He was weaned the day after he developed two teeth, one on each side of his jaw. He is reported to have enjoyed babyhood immensely.

He later trained at St Mary's Hospital Medical School, Paddington, London. He planned to specialise in adult medicine. However, within days of starting his first junior post in neonatal paediatrics at Harari Hospital in Rhodesia, it was obvious to him that he was doomed to lead a sleepless life with babies.

In search of higher technology he later returned to the UK and trained in paediatrics and neonatology at several prestigious centres, including the John Radcliffe Hospital, Oxford, and the Hospital for Sick Children, Great Ormond Street, London. After a fellowship in Neonatal Medicine at Denver Children's Hospital in the USA, he emigrated to Australia to become Director of Newborn Care at the Royal Hospital for Women, Paddington, Sydney.

He continues to practise in paediatrics and neonatology at the Royal Hospital for Women, St Margaret's Private Hospital and the Prince of Wales Children's Hospital, Sydney.

He was lucky enough to marry Tamara, who still copes with him, and they have two daughters, Georgina and Isabella.

YOU AND YOUR BABY

*Don't get bogged down in the
'right' way – there isn't one!
There's just you and your baby, a unique combination,
doing it together for the first time.*

This book was written as a guide for new mothers during their first months with their new baby. This second edition has been revised and expanded but it is still brief: now is a time for looking after the baby and trying to catch up on sleep, not for reading.

After looking after mothers and their babies for 20 years, the last 15 or so spent as Director of Newborn Care at the Royal Hospital for Women in Sydney, I have some idea of the questions that plague the new mother following birth. I also know of the incredible variety of answers she'll be subjected to if she asks them: some right, some wrong, and some laughable. This book has the best answers I know. If it's not enough, add a lot of common sense and a little trial and error.

It came as no surprise to those of us in the baby business that it was the babies who survived under the rubble caused by the Mexican earthquake, not, alas, their mothers. Babies are tough as old boots and come equipped with an amazing ability to survive adverse conditions. They are also equipped with the ability to teach their mothers all they need to know about bringing up babies. In order for mum to tune in to her little teacher, however, she must not fear making mistakes.

The only important error you can make is to seek answers from outside your relationship with your baby. That's when the trouble starts.

The reason isn't too subtle. Who doesn't find kittens cuddly? Even people who hate dogs like puppies, and so it is with babies. Human infants are magnetically attractive to most people and give satisfaction out of proportion to their size. This was a very useful mechanism in the days when many mothers did not survive childbirth and someone in the vicinity had to care enough to take over the baby. Now that good antenatal care and modern obstetrics have virtually eliminated the danger to the mother, the problem remains: everyone wants to get in on the act.

Everyone wants to 'help' you —that is, to persuade you to do it *their* way. Babies are so adaptable that virtually any way, as long as it's half reasonable, will work. So there are about fifty thousand ways to bring up a baby and they are all successful.

New mothers do sometimes feel in need of advice, particularly if they are having problems — with breastfeeding, for example. Don't seek advice from all and sundry: find someone you trust and listen only to that person. Conflicting advice is one of the greatest problems new mothers have. Be wary of advice. If it does not sound sensible, if it implies that babies are fragile objects that will break like eggshells unless handled in a particular way, if it suggests you need a degree in dietetics, paediatrics, hygiene and psychology to really understand — then ignore it!

Humanity is no worse off than the rest of the animal kingdom and nature has endowed all mothers with an instinctive knowledge of how to look after their baby. This knowledge does not lie in the intellect or in books, not even this one. It lies in the heart, the instinct and in the soft inner voice that says 'I should try this' or 'that advice doesn't sound right, I'll try this instead'. If you feel he's hungry, feed him. If he's not, he'll tell you and the next time he cries like that, you will know.

Don't get bogged down in the 'right' way — there isn't one! There's just you and your baby, a unique combination, doing it together for the first time.

Howard Chilton

During the course of this book I will always refer to mother as 'she' (I'm sure no-one will object) and to the baby as 'he' (some might). I am not sexist and I love girl babies too (I have two at home) but it's much less confusing than the 'he/she' alternative.

CHAPTER 1

BIRTH AND BEYOND

*Don't set too high a standard
for yourself or your baby.*

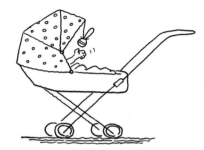

All the months of waiting are finally over. You've been to the antenatal classes, painted furniture, shopped for baby clothes and made endless plans. You have dreamed about the birth of your baby, and no doubt worried about how it would go, and then, after what seems like an eternity, the day finally arrives.

EXPECTATIONS

DON'T SET YOUR STANDARDS TOO HIGH

I once had a 'celebrity patient' whose baby got into minor trouble at birth by inhaling a bit of meconium. He puffed and panted and needed a bit of oxygen for a few hours. He remained in the special care nursery for three days and then joined his mother on the postnatal ward. Things did not go smoothly there either. There were feeding difficulties, sticky eyes, phototherapy for jaundice, a depressed mum — the works! Eventually everything sorted itself out and mother and baby went home in good shape.

Imagine the position of my eyebrows when, a couple of months later, I picked up a women's magazine of enormous circulation to see a feature on this lady's experience of childbirth. She was evidently Earth Mother herself, from the spiritual delivery to the gentle lying-in, from the smooth breastfeeding to the quiet satisfied baby at home. All was easy, fulfilling, natural and suffused with a warm, pink glow.

What a missed opportunity! If only she had told the vast readership the way it *really* was! How much more good it would have done. If only she had told of the agony as well as the ecstasy. The reality, not the fantasy of yet another idealised Hollywood role model that somehow we have come to think of as normal.

It is not surprising, therefore, that some mothers go through pregnancy and into delivery with their expectations just a little too high. They are expecting a quick, painless delivery, producing a perfect, beautiful, responsive infant who then breastfeeds like a natural. This does occur, and if it does, you're very lucky.

Alas, in reality things are usually not quite so picturesque. Contractions are a good deal more painful than some of you expect, although some are just lucky and have an easier time than others. Not only do pain thresholds vary greatly but so do the actual power of the contractions. Do not allow someone else to tell you how much pain you ought to be able to cope with. There is no pain easier to bear than somebody else's! Feeling guilty about the need for analgesia is too common in labour wards and birth centres and is so unnecessary. Labour should not be more painful than you can stand and your baby

can only benefit if you are comfortable enough to relax and enjoy the experience.

Some babies also decide that labour is too hard and insist upon being delivered by Caesarean section. In fact, this is up to 15 per cent of births in some urban populations. So you should consider in advance the idea that it might be necessary for you and your baby.

Following birth many babies prefer to spend the first day or so sleeping, and are reluctant to feed. He may virtually ignore his mother, who has worked so hard to bring him into the world.

Don't take it personally, just accept that labour and its aftermath may not be ideal and don't set too high a standard for yourself or your baby.

BREATHING

THE FIRST BREATH

How the system works

Within the womb the fetus floats in his ocean of amniotic fluid, supplied with oxygen and food from his mother's circulation through the placenta. His circulation bypasses the lungs through a couple of channels, one (called the *foramen ovale* or oval window) within the heart and the other (called the *ductus arteriosus* or arterial channel) outside. His lungs are filled with

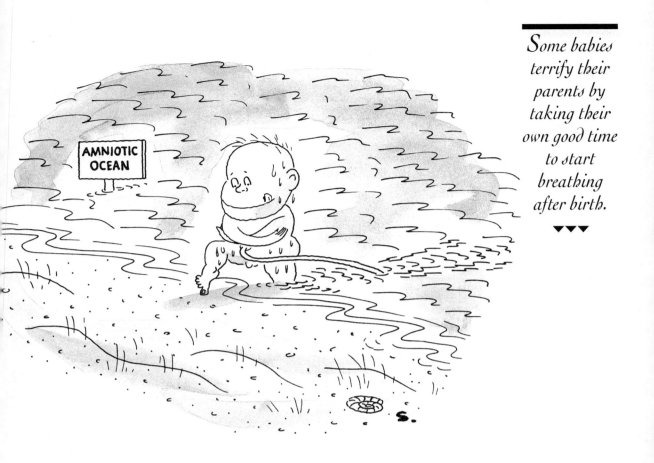

fluid and although he makes shallow breathing movements, his lungs are not used for absorbing oxygen.

On delivery many changes have to be made to adapt to living independently on dry land. The baby needs to get rid of about half a cupful (125 ml/4 fl oz) of fluid from his lungs, and this he does — usually rapidly. A third of it is squeezed out into his mouth when his chest is compressed by the birth canal (in a vaginal birth) and the rest is absorbed into his circulation following the first breath. In a

Caesarean delivery, all the fluid must be absorbed by his circulation. At the same time, under the combined stimulus of light, the cool air on his cheek, the different noise level and a rise in blood oxygen caused by his first breath, his circulation undergoes radical change.

With the first breath the channels which bypass the lungs constrict and close and the blood vessels in the lungs open up. This forces the blood through the lungs on each circulation, where it absorbs oxygen from the air waiting in the lungs from the breath. This oxygen is then carried to the body. Normally, this process is rapid and smooth and no help is required at the birth.

SLOW TO START

Some babies terrify their parents by taking their own good time to start breathing after birth. These babies may be grateful for a little assistance. A little gentle suction of the mouth and throat, usually to remove mucus, blood or fluid from the lungs, sometimes provides an extra stimulus to the breathing drive. If this is not enough the lungs can be inflated using a tight-fitting rubber mask and a ventilator bag. Most of the babies who require help will be stimulated by the action of the mask to continue breathing on their own. Now and again, especially if the babies are sick or the lungs are not mature, more resuscitation is required. A tube the size of a drinking straw may be inserted into the baby's windpipe (intubation) and the lungs inflated directly with the ventilation bag.

It is helpful to recognise how well designed babies are for delivery and how long they can manage without oxygen before any permanent harm ensues. A baby has to be totally without oxygen for at least 20 minutes before the brain may come to any permanent harm. Should the drive to start breathing on delivery be suppressed, the baby will be given help to get things going long before this occurs.

If your baby has been stretched beyond his ability to compensate, your paediatrician will be able to detect it within the first 12 to 24 hours. If your baby remains well during this time he has clearly coped with the situation.

WET LUNG

It has already been mentioned that a baby has about 125 ml (4 fl oz) of fluid in his lungs in the womb. Some babies are not very efficient at removing all this water from the lung after delivery. As there is less dry, useful lung tissue available, each breath is less efficient. Hence these babies need to breathe faster in order to get the right amount of air in and out of the lungs each minute. Therefore their respiratory rate, instead of being a slow and steady 40 a minute, may be a rather more rapid 60 or 70.

Another possible reason for rapid breathing after birth is the baby inhaling a little amniotic fluid before delivery. The result is the same. In medical parlance it is called 'transient tachypnoea' or 'wet lung' and is probably the commonest reason for otherwise healthy babies being admitted to an intensive care nursery after birth. In the nursery the baby is cared for, observed and occasionally given oxygen therapy. Usually the baby can get rid of the water in the lungs without any help within 24 hours and he can then return to his mother's side.

Unfortunately there's a downside. There is a third possible reason for babies breathing fast after birth. Babies are very vulnerable to infection and there is always the possibility of a lung infection acquired during the delivery. Luckily this problem is uncommon but it is impossible to immediately determine which few babies are infected. If there is *any* doubt at all, the baby's doctor takes no chances. Consequently many babies who breathe fast after birth will have a sample of blood taken and sent to the laboratory to be cultured for germs. If there is infection the germs will grow from this blood sample and a result can be determined in 48 hours. Meanwhile, the baby will be treated with antibiotics.

There is no question that this is the right way to approach this problem and avoid tragedy for the infected babies. Unfortunately, this means that many uninfected babies will receive antibiotics for 48 hours until the results of their blood cultures become known. We are not so concerned about the antibiotics in themselves (they are commonly used for babies and cause no problems) but we are concerned about the worry about a possible infection that we cause the parents, as well as the inconvenience of the intravenous drip.

If the cultures are negative then the antibiotics can safely be stopped straightaway. If they are positive then a full course of antibiotics has to be continued.

MECONIUM STAINING

There is one group of babies which is given special attention at delivery. In about 10 per cent of births, the amniotic fluid is stained with meconium (fetal stool). Meconium is a thick treacly substance that is harmless as long as it doesn't get deep into the baby's lungs. If it does, it acts as an irritant to the lining of the air passages and generally gums up the works. This can cause respiratory distress (breathlessness), pneumonia and other lung problems.

Consequently, when this baby's head emerges, his throat and nose are sucked out to remove any trace of meconium before he has had a chance to breathe. This will prevent him from inhaling it. If this meconium is difficult to remove he may be intubated at delivery to make sure that there is no meconium down his airway. This is good preventive medicine and will do him no harm.

Babies who inhale a little amniotic fluid usually get rid of it without any help within 24 hours.

▼▼▼

IMPORTANT INFECTIONS

There are two potentially nasty infections that may be present around the time of delivery that are worth discussing in some detail. One of these is the group B beta haemolytic streptococcus and the other is the herpes virus.

BETA STREP

The first germ, known as beta strep or GBS, resides in the birth canal of 5 to 30 per cent of women (it varies from area to area) and usually causes no problems. Its main importance is that if it is passed on to the baby at birth, 1 in 100 to 200 of them may become very sick. These babies may develop pneumonia, septicaemia and shock and some may well die, with little that neonatal medicine can do to help them. Of course, lesser degrees of the illness are possible and these babies may be rescued by antibiotics and intensive care.

Most obstetricians are now checking for the presence of this organism during the latter part of pregnancy by culturing a swab taken from the vagina. If it is found to be present it is possible to eliminate the organism by giving the mother a course of amoxycillin, or erythromycin if she is allergic to penicillin. However, it may return after a few weeks.

Large studies of maternity hospital populations have shown that if the presence of the organism is proved or suspected and the mother is given intravenous antibiotics (usually amoxycillin) early on in the labour, this reduces the likelihood of sickness in the babies to a very low level indeed.

When this organism causes infection in babies, often their first sign of illness after birth is respiratory distress (breathlessness). Consequently, most babies with this symptom are usually treated rapidly with antibiotics just to cover the possibility of infection, as was described in the earlier section about wet lung.

HERPES

A significant proportion of women nowadays carry the organism causing the second potentially nasty infection, the herpes virus. This causes recurrent ulcers in the genital tract especially around the vulva. These sores may last for three to five days and then heal completely. However, the recurrences may come and go for years. Another common condition caused by the herpes virus is the cold sore on the lips. This is a different species of the same virus but for all practical purposes can be viewed as the same. If babies are infected with herpes usually from

Beta strep (GBS) resides in the birth canal of 5 to 30 per cent of women and usually causes no problems.

▼▼▼

direct contact with an ulcer, it can be a devastating disease. They can suffer recurrent skin infections, brain damage or even die. Luckily such infection is quite rare despite the virus being common in mothers.

The reason for the rarity of the neonatal disease seems to be that the mother's antibodies travel to the baby through the placenta and protect him against catching the herpes infection at birth if an ulcer is present. These antibodies (like all other antibodies transferred from the mother) disappear from the baby's circulation in the first three to six months following delivery. However, they work very well at birth which is the time when he is most likely to be in contact with any recurrent herpetic ulcers his mother may have in the birth canal.

A few years ago obstetricians were so frightened of the baby catching herpes from a recurrent ulcer in his mother that a Caesarean section was performed if one was present. We now know that the danger is extremely low, so vaginal delivery is safe.

Of course the baby is still extremely vulnerable if the delivery occurs when his mother is having her very first attack of herpes ulcers — that is, it is his mother's 'primary' infection. Under this circumstance, the mother has no antibodies to give the baby protection and up to half of these babies will catch the infection.

Another important point is that, as described earlier, the herpes antibodies in the baby's circulation will wear out after a few months, thus making the baby vulnerable to the herpes virus. So later on, during an attack, it is most important that careful hygiene be maintained, hands washed carefully and care taken not to put the baby in contact with the ulcers.

Similarly, if his mother has not had herpes, then there are no antibodies and the baby is very vulnerable to catching the virus. Hence the cold sores on the lips of his father, friends and relations can be a real danger. Indeed this is the commonest source of the virus in babies who catch herpes. It is most important that active cold sores be kept away from the baby.

OTHERS

There are other organisms which reside in the birth canal that can cause infections of the baby if they are present at the time of birth. There are two common sexually-transmitted germs which can either cause overt infection or lie dormant on the cervix or in the vagina and still cause problems for the baby. Gonorrhoea can cause septicaemia and severe eye infection and chlamydia can cause eye and lung infection.

If you think there is a possibility you may have been exposed to

Despite the herpes virus being common in mothers, the infection is quite rare in babies.

either gonorrhoea or chlamydia, let your doctor know so you can be tested.

Genital warts usually don't infect babies, although the occasional case has been reported.

The commonest infection in the vagina during pregnancy is thrush, which causes few, if any, problems in the baby. Though some babies may get a mild infection in their mouth, there are many other sources of the fungus besides their mother.

Finally, if you are a carrier of the hepatitis B virus, your baby s vulnerable. Nowadays he can be completely protected by getting both active and passive immunisation. An injection of an antibody (HBIG or hepatitis B immunoglobulin) soon after birth will protect him for the first few weeks. Also, he should be given the first of a course of hepatitis B vaccine injections. He will need another after one month and a third at six months to complete the course.

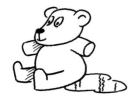

CHAPTER 2

THE SEAL OF APPROVAL

Birthright and birthrite:
a thorough, competent physical examination
of the newborn infant.

Every newborn infant should have a thorough physical examination early on in his life. Such examinations are designed to detect the difficulties of adapting to life outside the womb and any congenital abnormalities or illnesses. During his stay in hospital the baby will usually have at least two or three physical examinations.

IN THE DELIVERY ROOM

As soon as a baby is born he will be examined to assess any difficulty he may be encountering converting from a dependent life inside the womb, relying on the placenta for food and oxygen, to an independent life outside, using the lungs to obtain oxygen. This examination will also find any important congenital abnormalities that need immediate management and treatment. The doctor or midwife can then assure his terrified parents that they can stop worrying!

It is at this time that the Apgar score is done. Five physical signs of the baby are scored either 0, 1 or 2 to assess how well he's adapting to life outside the womb and whether he has been affected by delivery. The baby is assessed at one minute after birth and again at five minutes after birth.

When the baby has settled down and is warm, dry and comfortable, a paediatrician will examine him thoroughly.

APGAR SCORE
PERFORMED AT ONE AND FIVE MINUTES AFTER DELIVERY

PHYSICAL SIGNS	SCORE 0	SCORE 1	SCORE 2
Heart rate	Absent	Less than 100	More than 100
Respiratory effort	Absent	Slow and irregular	Good and regular
Muscle tone	Limp	Some flexion of limbs	Active motion
Colour	Blue	Pink body, blue extremeties	Completely pink
Reflex response	Nil	Grimace	Cough or sneeze to nasal catheter

THE NEWBORN BABY

Newborns often worry their parents by their sometimes strange appearance. Most of these odd characteristics are quite normal and will disappear sooner or later.

- swollen eyes
- throbbing fontanelle
- enlarged genitals
- rash of white spots over face
- changes in skin colour
- a coating of greasy white vernix
- fine hair over the back and shoulders called lanugo
- misshapen head, generally due to compression in the birth canal
- instrument marks (if there was a forceps delivery)
- turned-in feet
- bowed legs
- small, rather receding chin
- blue hands and feet
- swollen nipples
- ingrowing toenails
- rubbery lumps under the skin of the cheekbones and jaw
- swelling or bruising on the head as a result of labour
- red marks over the eyelids, nose and back of neck

Full physical examination

A paediatrician can obtain lots of information about the baby merely by observing him. Following this general look a more specific examination can be conducted.

Observation

Posture. The baby usually lies in a relaxed posture with arms by his sides, elbows bent, hips and knees flexed. His body is straight with his head on one side.

Colour. His colour is generally pink in Caucasian and Asian babies and rather darker in Negroid babies, although his hands and feet may be blue and cool for the first few days. After two or three days his colour may become slightly yellowish as the normal jaundice occurs.

Breathing. He breathes quietly at a rate of about 40 breaths a minute but may also have the pattern of alternate panting and shallow breathing which is normal for the first three months of life.

Facial appearance. His face is examined to see whether it conforms to a normal appearance (if it seems a little unusual the paediatrician will usually have a look at dad before saying so!).

Skin

Maturity

The thickness of the skin relates to the baby's maturity. A baby born early has fine, pink, delicate skin whereas the skin of a postmature baby (a baby born two weeks or more after term) has a pale, scaly, parchment-like appearance. White, greasy material, called vernix, may be present (especially in the creases), in all babies but particularly in those born a week or two early.

Birthmarks

Most babies have got so-called 'stork-bites' which are flat red birthmarks over the eyelids, bridge of the nose and back of the neck. The ones on the face disappear over the first year or so.

'Mongolian spots' are irregular areas of deep blue pigmentation usually found above or around the buttocks. They occur in all races but especially in Asians and they mostly fade over the first few years.

More unusual are strawberry marks, which disappear without treatment before the age of five, and port-wine stains, which don't disappear unless they are treated, usually with laser therapy.

Milia

These little white spots (like millet seeds — hence the name) are due to distended sweat glands and are mostly seen over the cheeks, chin

Some babies have bruises and other marks from delivery. Have no fear, within a couple of days most of the marks will be gone.

▼▼▼

and nose. They are probably caused by the effect of hormones from the placenta on the developing sweat gland. Don't worry about them, even if they increase in number, as they disappear after the first few weeks.

Other marks

Some babies have bruises and other marks from the delivery, especially on their heads and faces. Have no fear, babies are designed beautifully for what they have to go through (you!) and heal very rapidly. Within a couple of days most of the marks will have gone.

Don't get upset about forceps marks. This instrument has got a bad name quite unfairly. A forceps delivery is actually preferred by many paediatricians for premature babies. The forceps act as a protective cage around the soft skull. Used properly, they do good, not harm. They are primarily used to guide the head of the baby through the lower part of the mother's pelvis if progress is slow or the head is in the wrong position or the mother is too tired to push.

THE HEAD

The paediatrician will measure the head circumference and feel the fontanelle and the edges of the skull bones.

Head shape

Babies are a bit like toothpaste in their ability to fit through tight places. Following delivery, particularly when the birth canal is narrow, the baby's head may be elongated and misshapen. This is very common and my only advice is to stop worrying and delay taking the first baby photographs.

Babies are designed very well for the journey down the birth canal. In particular, the skull bones (of which there are four over the vault of the head) are not fused and can override each other to allow the head to pass down a narrow birth canal. This overriding, or molding, may be detected as thickening over the midline or above the ears following delivery. It disappears in the first few days and no harm can come to the brain underneath.

The head may also develop caput, which is a boggy, irregular swelling of the soft tissues of the skull, again due to compression by the birth canal during labour.

The bone may also become swollen. Bone has a membrane stuck firmly down to its surface, and during delivery, if the flat skull bone is flexed a little, this membrane may split off and there may be

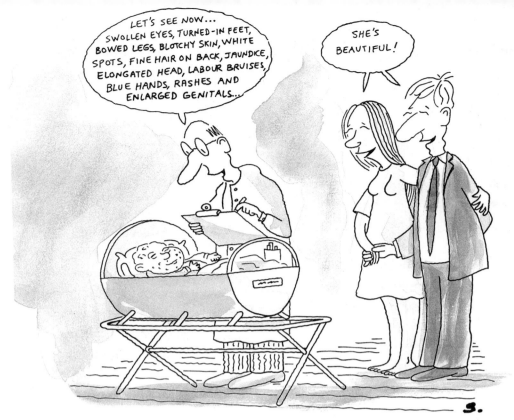

bleeding underneath it. This gives a soft boggy swelling called a cephal-haematoma, which takes a few weeks to disappear. In 20 per cent of cases, however, the swelling turns to bone and the skull shape remodels over a longer period of time, but it does disappear eventually.

The fontanelle

This is a diamond-shaped soft spot at the top of the head, which is easily indented with the finger. Despite its apparent vulnerability, it is a very thick, tough membrane and there is no danger at all of injuring your baby with normal handling. It often gets a little larger in the first few months before closing between the ages of 9 and 18 months.

You may notice that it sometimes pulsates with the heartbeat: this is normal. It also bulges when the baby cries or strains. This is invariably normal if the bulging goes away when the baby stops screaming or is sat upright. Conversely, sitting babies up will either make their fontanelle flat or sunken. Again, this is not a problem. You may have heard that a sunken fontanelle can be related to dehydration and, indeed, that is an important sign. However, it is a very late sign of it and the dehydra-tion would have to be severe. So if the baby is wetting more than three nappies a day and isn't obviously ill and dry then don't worry. It's not a physical sign that means anything on its own.

Despite its apparent vulnerability, the fontanelle is a very thick, tough membrane.

▼▼▼

THE EYES

These are usually clear, blue grey or brown. Their final colour may not be obvious until the baby is about a year old. Small spots of blood within the white of the eye are very common and are due to the bursting of capillaries from the compression during labour. They are completely harmless and disappear in a week or so. An intermittent squint is normal, especially when the baby feeds, and unless it is constant, there is no cause for concern. Parents should realise that their babies see clearly from birth.

THE MOUTH

Small white cysts are frequently seen along the gum margins and on the hard palate, especially in the midline. They can be mistaken for thrush, are of no consequence and will soon disappear without treatment.

THE CHEST

Breast enlargement is seen in many infants and is of no significance. Sometimes there is a secretion of milky substance due to the stimulating effect of the hormones from the placenta. It is hardly necessary to examine the lungs with a stethoscope as a normal respiratory rate is by far the most sensitive index. Parents often notice a solid lump in the midline just below the breast-bone (sternum) at the top of the abdomen in their baby. This is the xiphisternum — the extension to the sternum made of cartilage. It is normal.

THE HEART

The normal heart rate is usually between 100 and 140 beats per minute. The heart is also checked with a stethoscope for the sound of a murmur. Most murmurs picked up in the first few days are due either to delay in the circulation changing from that of a fetus to that of a newborn, or to the presence of tiny holes between the two main pumping chambers in the heart. Both of these problems right themselves within a short time and are harmless.

THE ABDOMEN

The doctor examines the abdomen to ensure the liver, spleen and kidneys are normal and also feels for any abnormal lumps or masses. The umbilicus contains three vessels (one vein and two arteries). Occasionally an umbilical hernia may be present (see the later section on Umbilical Hernia, pages 87-88, for more details). This is of no significance as it rarely requires surgery and disappears by itself in time, usually by the age of five.

At the junction of the abdomen and the thighs, the main (femoral) arteries to the legs can be felt with the fingertips. A normal pulse will show there is no narrowing of the artery higher up.

THE GENITALS

These will be inspected carefully for any abnormalities. In boys, both testes are in the scrotum. Cold hands, however, may make them disappear temporarily as there is a reflex which pulls them up out of sight. Occasionally the testes are held up on their journey down from the abdomen. They are then termed undescended. Ninety per cent of these will descend on their own in the first year; the rest may require surgery to bring one or both into the scrotum.

In girls, the vulva looks rather swollen and red in comparison to later life. Occasionally the labia minora (inner lips) protrude between the labia majora (outer lips). This is normal in the term baby and common in even the slightly premature. Mucus tags and occasionally bleeding may be seen at the opening of the vagina. Both occur because of stimulation from hormones from the placenta and neither is of any significance.

THE HIPS

The hip joints are examined for clicks (which are quite common, and harmless, in the newborn) or dislocation. Your doctor will examine the baby's hips again before you and your baby are discharged from the hospital. (See the section on Congenital Dislocation of Hips, pages 40-43, for more details.)

THE LEGS AND FEET

It is normal for babies to have bow legs. The slight curvature of the tibia is caused by their posture inside the womb. Most babies hold their feet turned inwards while in the womb and this may continue to be obvious for a few weeks after delivery. Occasionally this is called 'postural talipes' by some but this is not the talipes of club foot. If the foot can be held at right angles to the leg with the sole flat, then it is a normal ankle joint.

THE BACK

The doctor will check the spine to see that it is straight and has no faults. Very commonly there is a dimple at the base of the spine. This is quite normal and will grow out with time. The doctor will also check the anus to see that it is open.

It is normal for babies to have bow legs.

▼▼▼

THE NERVOUS SYSTEM

SIGHT AND HEARING

Throughout the examination, the posture, muscle tone, responses, moods, movements and cry of the baby are all observed and noted. He can be seen to turn to and gaze at light and will often stare fixedly at a face.

Hearing is somewhat more difficult to test in the first few days as the baby is very tolerant of loud noises. Remember, he has just emerged from the noisy environment of the womb, with his mother's aorta, the main artery of her body, banging away centimetres from his ear, her bowels gurgling and her bladder filling and emptying. However, he will usually respond to a clap or a loud noise if you catch him in the right mood.

REFLEXES

His reflexes will be tested. A baby is born with a number of automatic reactions to changes in his position or environment called 'primitive' reflexes. These are seen as a hangover from an early stage of human evolution. These reflexes

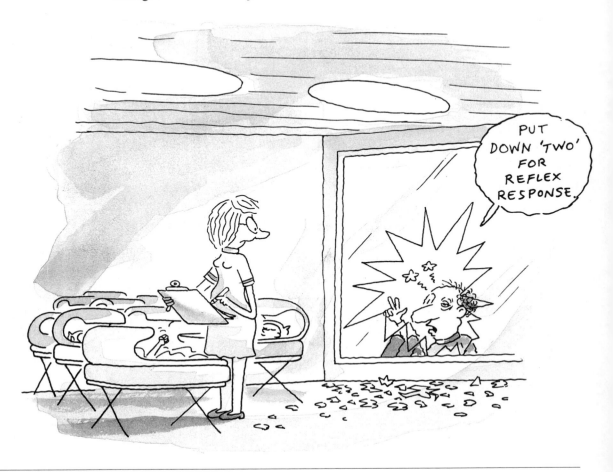

disappear over the first weeks and months and their disappearance indicates normal development of the baby's nervous system.

Especially obvious is his 'startle' (Moro) reflex. If the baby's chin is positioned on his chest and his head is allowed to fall back, he will respond by flinging his arms out as if to grab at something. He will then move them in an arc towards the midline of his chest. At the same time he will open his eyes wide, look unhappy, and may start to cry. A test of the Moro reflex is a good check of the baby's muscle tone. The reflex disappears gradually over the first two to three months.

Another reflex is his 'grasp' reflex. If you tickle his palm he will grip your finger. In fact, he will automatically close his hand if something is placed in his palm. This reflex is so strong that he can actually support his body weight grasping two of your fingers. His toes will also flex in response to a similar stimulus to the sole of the foot.

If you brush your baby's cheek on one side he will turn his head in that direction. This is called the rooting reflex, and will ensure that he will root for the nipple when his cheek brushes against his mother's breast.

Proud parents often like to demonstrate their baby's 'walking' reflex. A baby, held in the standing position with feet on a flat surface,

will make somewhat clumsy walking movements forward. This reflex disappears at about the age of four weeks.

The 'stepping' reflex is another interesting one. By bringing the baby's shin in contact with the edge of a flat surface, the leg will be raised to step over it as though he were climbing a staircase.

The 'Galant' reflex can be elicited by holding the baby over one hand, back towards you. By stimulating the lumbar region, for instance with a gentle scratch, the baby will curve his bottom towards the side of the stimulus.

DISCHARGE EXAMINATION

Just before your baby goes home your doctor will carry out a final examination. This is to check the following things:

- The heart is checked to be sure no murmurs have emerged since the first examination. Because the baby's circulation is making great changes in these first few days some murmurs take a few days to develop.
- The head circumference is remeasured now that most of the molding has disappeared.
- The umbilical cord is checked for infection, and to make sure that

A baby is born with a number of automatic reactions to changes in his position or environment. These reactions are called 'primitive' reflexes.

▼▼▼

the normal process of drying and separation is occurring.

- The baby's eyes are checked for 'stickiness', and, if necessary, tear duct massage is taught to the mother.
- The skin is examined for any rashes or pustules.
- The hips are rechecked just to be on the safe side. Those hips whose ligaments were marginally lax on the first day should now be much firmer in their sockets and, if so, can be safely left alone but carefully followed up.
- The feeding is assessed to see if it is going well. The baby is usually weighed — though at this stage whether or not there is any gain doesn't mean much.

Any questions you have can be answered. Now is the time to clear up any conflicting advice you may have been given, and to find out how to get help if things start to worry you after you go home. Don't waste the opportunity! On the next page are some of the questions most frequently asked.

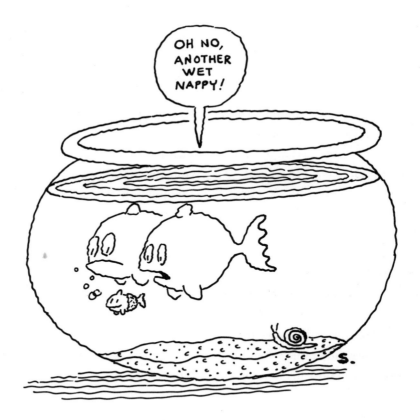

QUESTIONS AND ANSWERS

Being a first-time mother is by definition a new experience, full of tasks to be learned and problems to be solved. In the light of this, there is no such thing as a stupid question. Use these questions as a basis for your own list, writing down any others as they occur to you.

Q.If he vomits some of his feed, should I top him up again?

A.That depends on him. If he appears willing to suck, top him up and if he does not seem to mind, wait for him to demand before putting him back on the breast.

Q.Should I clean my baby's ears? Is there a safe way to do it?

A.It is not a good idea to immerse your baby's ears in water as the canal is difficult to dry and can get infected. Clean only the part of the ear that you can see. Do not poke anything rigid into the ear canal.

Q.When should I take him to see the health centre nurse?

A.First babies should probably go weekly to start with until weight gain is established, then as often as you wish. For subsequent babies, fortnightly visits are usually enough.

Q.If my baby gets a rash, should I go on bathing him, and with what?

A.Don't use soap on the affected area. Use a nonsoap cleanser or pine tar solution in his bath. It's not necessary to bathe him every day. First babies get bathed every day, second babies alternate days and fourth babies twice a week!

Q.How do I know when my baby has had enough at a feed?

A.He will stop sucking and may fall asleep (but not necessarily). If he does, don't wake him by burping him, put him down in his cot.

Q.How many wet nappies should I expect my baby to have each day?

A.Babies who are being well fed may have between five to twelve wet nappies a day. If he has only two, let your doctor or midwife know.

Q.How do I handle the stump of his umbilical cord? Will it bleed? When and how will it heal up and fall off?

A.Remember that your baby cannot feel pain from his umbilical cord so handling it will cause him no discomfort. Give it a gentle tug when cleaning it to get down into the gutter. Cords often bleed a little in the days after birth but it is usually only backflow from the clotted veins within the cord and is of no significance. The umbilical cord heals up by becoming gummy and separating at the base. This process can take between four days and six weeks.

Q.Should I clean the baby's genital area and how? Should I draw back the foreskin or should I leave it alone?

A.Do not draw back the foreskin until it has separated from the glans underneath when it will become easier to retract. This may take one year or more. Take your lead from your little boy; he will play with it in his bath and show you how far back it can comfortably be retracted. For little girls, gentle spreading of the outer lips and drawing a wet cotton-wool ball from front to back within the vulva is often necessary. The vagina is self-cleaning.

SMALL BABIES

Babies who weigh less than 2.5 kg (5½ lbs) at birth are defined as small. Smallness can be due to several reasons.

The baby's parents may be small. In this case the baby would behave and have the same needs as any other full-term baby.

The baby may be premature. Such a baby may have immaturity of some important functions, resulting in poor sucking and feeding, respiratory difficulty, a tendency to get cold easily or for the blood sugar level to drop, and general lethargy.

The baby may be 'small for dates'. This baby is more mature than his weight implies but he is undernourished, usually because the placenta, and hence food transferral from his mother, did not function well in the final weeks.

Babies in the last two groups are given extra attention until they are stable and functioning as a larger baby might. Obviously, if the babies are very small, unstable or require special care for any reason, they are admitted to a neonatal intensive care unit. Their management is beyond the scope of this book; however, suffice it to say that the vast majority of babies admitted to such units do very well and, if premature, will be home by the time they are 38 weeks gestation.

OBSERVATIONS

Small babies who are, however, big enough to stay with their mother in the postnatal ward are checked regularly, with observations of respiratory rate, heart rate and temperature every four hours. They also have regular heel-prick tests with Dextrostix or BM sticks to measure the blood sugar level.

MANAGEMENT

If the baby is a week or so premature (that is, 35 to 36 weeks gestation) the mother can expect feeding to take a little longer to establish, as the suck reflex may not be at full strength for a few days. It can require a lot of patience and determination to stick to breastfeeding with some of the slower ones.

In contrast, the 'small for dates' baby may have a voracious appetite and work hard to put on the weight he feels is his birthright — at his poor mother's expense. Again, patience!

When his weight catches up (usually within the first three months) he'll suddenly settle down to a more relaxed schedule.

It is worth remembering that these babies have poor stores of energy for the first few days. This means that an eye must be kept on their blood sugar level until it is stable. This is easily monitored with regular checks of heel-prick blood.

They may also require complementary feeds of formula if they are too small to wait for the arrival of the breast milk in two to three days. In addition, their temperature must be checked regularly as babies can chill easily when inadequately dressed in a cool environment.

Small babies should be immunised at the usual time — from their birthdate, NOT corrected for their prematurity.

THE EMPTY-HANDED MOTHER

It is pretty depressing if your baby needs to be in the special care nursery instead of by your side. Quite apart from the anxiety, there is often a feeling that you have let him down because you cannot meet all of his needs by yourself and that in some way your bonding with your baby will suffer (properly managed, it will not).

Special care nurseries seem to evoke different responses in different parents. Some find the technology reassuring: they feel that all the equipment is really making their baby better. Others are just terrified that their baby needs to be looked after in an environment that seems more suitable for an astronaut than their precious baby.

You will be encouraged to spend as much time as possible with your baby and if this feels comfortable, do it. If, on the other hand, sitting by him terrifies and panics you, do not feel compelled to do so. After a few days you will feel comfortable enough to stay with him for longer and longer periods. There are no hard and fast rules.

Many parents, especially mothers, go through a brief period much like grieving if their baby has a problem after birth. They grieve for the loss of the perfection they imagined during the pregnancy. They may feel disappointment and anger, as well as sadness and anxiety, as they struggle to adjust. These powerful emotions are either directed inwardly, as guilt, or outwardly, as anger towards the partner, the doctors and nurses and even the baby.

Like every other part of the body, our mind also has to heal when it has been injured, and these emotions are a part of the healing process. Accept them for what they are — a painful but important pathway to feeling better. They will pass and, for the vast majority of mothers, be replaced by joy as the healthy baby is placed in her arms.

Vitamin K

Soon after your baby is born, he will be
offered an injection of vitamin K.
This practice is pretty universal, and for good reason.

Until 30 years ago there was an important, common and potentially lethal condition of babies called 'haemorrhagic disease of the newborn' which affected up to 1.5 per cent of babies. Typically, a few days after delivery, the baby's clotting system would cease to work efficiently, and bleeding, often severe, would occur from the umbilical cord or the bowel. He would often recover spontaneously if the haemorrhage was minor but if it was brisk he could rapidly develop shock caused by the loss of blood, and, unless treated, could die. The treatment was transfusion and vitamin K.

WHAT DOES VITAMIN K DO?

The blood-clotting system of the body is based on a complex series of reactions between many proteins and chemicals called clotting factors. Many of these require vitamin K for their activation and without it poor coagulation (clotting) results. When this was realised, the use of a routine injection of vitamin K after birth became commonplace and the disease virtually disappeared.

That is, until the last ten years or so. Since then there have been a growing number of reports of a new and deadlier form of haemorrhagic disease. This form occurs later, about four to six weeks after delivery and the bleeding is often in the brain, with serious consequences. The babies in these recent reports have two things in common. Firstly, they did not receive vitamin K after birth, and secondly, they were all exclusively breastfed.

Studies have shown that many healthy babies born at full term have only marginally satisfactory stores of vitamin K. By the third day of life, as they start to grow, vitamin K deficiency can emerge. Giving vitamin K to the mother before delivery does not seem to help, as it passes across the placenta poorly. Anyway, many mothers have relatively low levels of vitamin K in their blood towards the end of their pregnancy.

We also know that breast milk contains only very small amounts of vitamin K. Cow's milk and commercial infant formula have very much higher levels than breast milk (up to ten times as much). If a nursing mother is supplied with adequate vitamin K in her diet, a little will appear in her milk and be absorbed by the baby, but nowhere near enough to prevent haemorrhagic disease. If you are breast-feeding it is a good idea to eat some fresh green leafy vegetables every day, as these are a rich source of this important vitamin.

WHY HAS HAEMORRHAGIC DISEASE REAPPEARED?

There are probably two reasons. Firstly, with the recent movement against technology in birthing and the recent 'cancer' scare (discussed below) there are some babies whose parents refuse the vitamin K offered to every newborn baby. Secondly, a few years ago most babies received at least a little formula or cow's milk as supplement, even when fully breastfed and this small amount was enough to boost the baby's vitamin K level and avoid deficiency. Nowadays, anxiety (largely misplaced) about cow's milk allergy means it is more likely that he will receive no such supplement.

THE ADMINISTRATION OF VITAMIN K

For over 20 years most of the developed world has been using an injection of 1 mg of vitamin K given at birth to the baby. This completely eliminated haemorrhagic disease of the newborn and was apparently without any side effects or danger.

Then in 1992 a study from England was published which showed that there was a remote possibility that this injection might double the risk of childhood cancer in those who received it. There did not seem to be any added risk for those babies who received vitamin K by mouth. There were many scientific problems with this study. The article reported that the authors had gone back over the records of a group of babies who were born some 20 years before and who had received an injection of vitamin K. The authors had tried to compare them with a similar group of babies who did not receive vitamin K or received it orally. Even the authors of the study pointed out the shortcomings of their work.

In addition, there is virtually no logical basis for belief that the conclusion is true. There is very little information that vitamin K has any relationship to anything other than blood-clotting, least of all cancer production. Also 'cancer' is not a single disease and as the cancers reviewed were of many different types, it is hard to believe there is a connection between them, when they actually represent unrelated diseases. No other carcinogen, not even nuclear bombs, produces cancer in so many different tissues.

We must always remember that in studies like this 'nonsense correlations' can occur. For instance it could probably be shown that

Breast milk contains only very small amounts of Vitamin K. Cow's milk & commercial infant formula have higher levels.

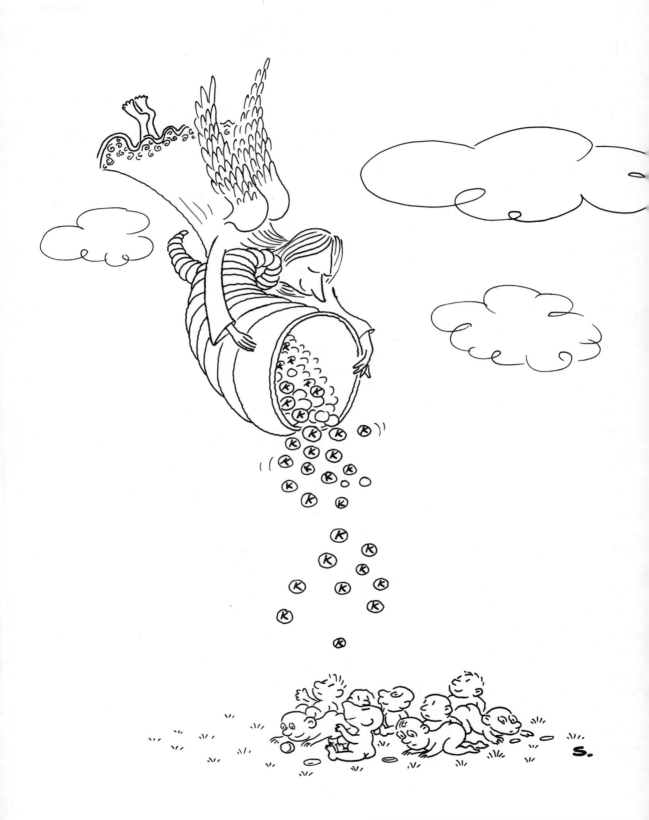

most middle-aged men who have coronary heart disease own a colour television, but nobody would blame the TV for their chest pain!

However, the most powerful argument against the conclusion resides in the leukaemia statistics from countries that have used the injection for 20 years or so. Nowhere has the incidence of that disease changed at all. It has stayed at a level of about four per million (ages 0 to 4 years), and seven per million (5 to 9 years) since the late 1940s. This is shown by statistics from the USA, the UK and elsewhere, including New South Wales, Australia. Most persuasive and most exhaustive was the study done in Sweden in response to the original English study. They looked at the data from 1.3 million infants born over a 16-year period, of whom 1 million were given vitamin K by injection, and the rest were given it orally. They were unable to find any difference in cancer or leukaemia statistics. The information gathered was beautifully complete and, in the opinion of most authorities, has exonerated the injection completely.

When the uproar started there was a swing away from injection to oral vitamin K in some countries. Unfortunately, the oral form at present needs at least three separate doses to be given for it to be as reliable as the injection. Not un-expectedly, some cases of haem-orrhagic disease have reappeared, with some totally unnecessary deaths.

Some authorities suggest that even if the conclusions are untrue, it is a good idea that the vitamin be given orally as a routine. They recommend that babies receive 1 mg of vitamin K orally on day one, day four and again at four weeks of age. This is nearly as reliable as the injection and will do until such time as an oral preparation is available which is as effective given as a single injection dose (which should be fairly soon). The danger is, of course, that if all three doses are not taken there is a real risk of the baby developing haemorrhagic disease.

Other authorities, such as the American Academy of Pediatrics (which, I might add, belongs to the most litigious and cancer-phobic society on earth), are reassured by the arguments above and suggest no change to present practice.

The essence of the discussion is to minimise the risk for our babies. There is little doubt, now that the shouting and arm-waving have stopped and reliable information has been obtained, that an injection of vitamin K is the safest way for your baby to be protected.

There is little doubt that the injection of Vitamin K is the safest way for your baby to be protected.

▼▼▼

CHAPTER 3

EARLY DAYS

*It takes time to fall in love
with your baby.*

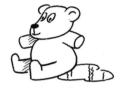

It is important to remember, when we read so much about what can go wrong during pregnancy and childbirth, that most babies are born free of problems. Occasionally there may be some early difficulties, most of which will be quite quickly resolved.

BONDING

A lot has been said and written about bonding over the last several years which seems to imply that it is a straightforward mechanism. This approach says that if you don't see and hold your baby immediately on delivery, always have him in sight and breastfeed him, then your relationship may never recover!

This black and white approach may be appropriate for lower animals like rats, sheep and goats, but for such a complex organism as a human being it is manifestly untrue. Not only does it defy common sense (and what we all know about adopting parents), but careful

scientific studies have shown that our system is far more complex than this. Humans possess great flexibility and enormous ability to cope with adverse circumstances at birth and after.

However, that is not to say that it's all rubbish. If the mother has a comfortable delivery, comes from a stable family, is conscious during her baby's birth, the delivery lives up to her expectations and is not too painful, she breastfeeds the baby early and has him in her room with her in the postnatal period, this mother will probably have an easier time falling in love with her baby and feeling confident about meeting his needs after she goes home.

If she misses any of those factors it will make either no, or very little, difference to her abilities in the end but it is possible she could have more difficulty getting to feel comfortable with her baby. That is, the instincts to look after her baby may flow less easily from her and the process may take a little longer.

It is also unrewarding to compare, as some experts have, the bonding behaviour of, say, sheep with humans and try to derive reasonable conclusions that apply to human mothers and their babies. For instance, a mother ewe bonds instantly with her newborn lamb at birth and that bond can easily be disrupted if it is not allowed to occur straight after delivery.

Why should biology arrange one system for sheep and another for humans? Sheep all deliver their lambs at the same time. Imagine 300 ewes and 300 lambs all milling around in a field. If ewe and lamb did not immediately attach to each other there could be a lot of confusion in that paddock at feedtime.

Humans in prehistoric times lived in small groups — perhaps 10 or 15 in number. There would only be two or three babies at the most in any group and they would have been delivered at different times. This would give the mothers ample opportunity to get to know their own baby — and the babies would also be shared to some degree with the other women in the group.

Leboyer — fact or fad? The great fashion for Leboyer deliveries was based upon the belief that a quiet nonclinical atmosphere is preferable at the delivery, which is true, and that the baby's relationship with his parents, his behaviour and security would be improved in the long term, which is not true. It has been demonstrated in carefully-controlled studies that, after one year, there is no discernible difference between the babies born of Leboyer deliveries and the babies born of routine deliveries.

Don't misunderstand me. Factors which enhance bonding are excellent and should be encouraged because they may make the task of getting to love your baby easier. But if you miss any of them because, for instance, you have a general anaesthetic for a Caesarean section, or your baby has to spend 24 hours in the special care unit, or you decide to bottle-feed for whatever reason, don't worry — your bond will be just as strong, and 'bond' is the right word. You're stuck for life.

IT TAKES TIME TO FALL IN LOVE WITH YOUR BABY

This message was on a banner draped across the nursery in the hospital of the famous English paediatrician, Sir Hugh Jolly. He recognised how many mothers worried that there they were, five days after the birth, and the baby was still 'just a baby'. No pink glow, no rending hearts, he's just a blob — and a noisy one at that. If you feel like that about your baby, be reassured that many other mothers feel just the same — and they too hate to admit the way they feel.

A study showed that over 30 per cent of mothers still felt indifferent towards their babies after several days, and some mothers took over a month before they felt comfortable with their baby.

▼▼▼

Bonding is the right word — your're stuck for life.

▼▼▼

*Babies are
incredibly
responsive to
things around
them in the
first few days
after birth.*

▼▼▼

A study showed that over 30 per cent of mothers still felt indifferent towards their babies after several days, and some mothers took over a month before they felt comfortable with their baby. We are all different. We all deal with changes and accept new people into our lives at a different pace and in different ways. Give it at least three months before you start to worry. Then if you can't stand him because he looks like your mother-in-law, perhaps you had better talk it over with your doctor who will put you in touch with people who can help you.

RESPONSIVENESS

'WHEN WILL MY BABY BE ABLE TO SEE?'

It is sad how many parents don't realise how incredibly responsive their baby is to things around him in the first few days and weeks after birth.

First and foremost, don't believe those people who tell you babies can't see for weeks. They see clearly. They are, however, a little short-sighted, focusing best at a distance of about 20 cm (8 in). Not only do they see well, but within just a few minutes of delivery, babies will often show a 'face-searching' reflex. Babies actually have a preference for looking at the human face rather than other patterns or objects. Many will stare at mother or father for long periods in the early hours after birth — a sure-fire way to melt a heart. The baby also learns to recognise his mother's smell within a few days of birth and has definite taste preference. He certainly responds positively to touch, enjoying stroking and relishing skin-to-skin contact.

Most fascinating is the fact that he has the ability to imitate a facial expression shown him. Get him in a quiet, alert mood and try sticking out your tongue to him. Within just a few days of birth he will try to stick out his tongue too.

And to think that it wasn't so long ago that people thought babies were just blobs for the first few weeks! Far from it — your baby is a real person right from day one.

FIRST-DAY MUCUS

Many babies vomit a lot of mucus in the first 24 to 48 hours. The mucus is produced by the stomach lining as a reaction to delivery. It may be continually produced in excess for a day or two, so washing out the stomach with a tube does no good. The mucus, which may be bloodstained, sometimes also makes the baby reluctant to feed.

This mucus is also the commonest cause of 'blue turns' during this period. It can be very thick, like

*Your baby is
a real person
right from
day one.*

▼▼▼

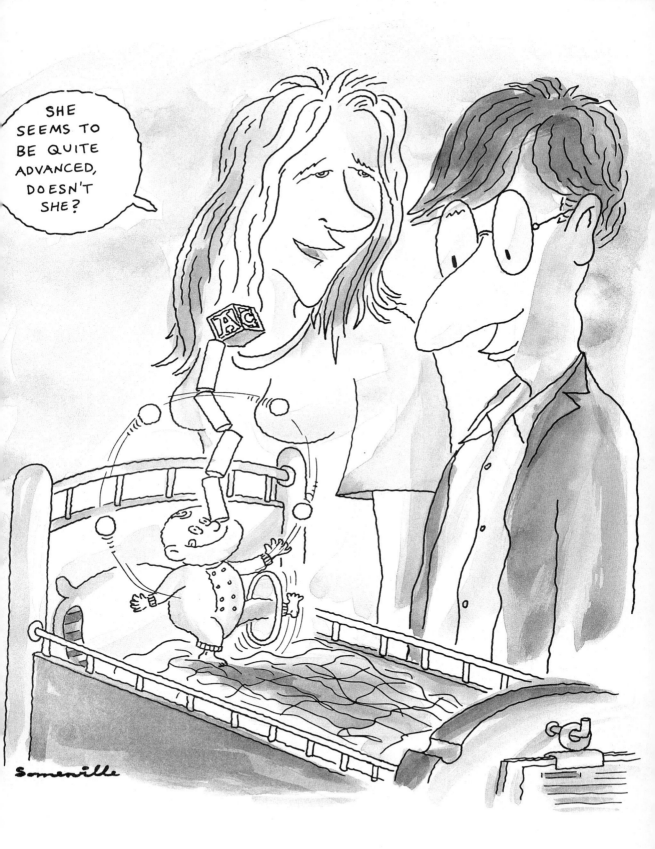

treacle, and can cause temporary obstruction to the baby's breathing. This usually gives mothers quite a fright but it is important to remember that the baby's breathing drive and his cough reflex are very powerful and he will be able to cough the obstruction out of the way without help. There is no need for any special treatment, but tipping the baby onto his side and patting his back can't do any harm.

Massaging the tear duct gently is the ideal treatment for sticky eyes.

STICKY EYES

About 15 per cent of babies develop sticky eyes within a few days of birth. One or both eyes start to discharge mucus or pus from under the lids. It can be so profuse as to gum the lids together, especially after the baby has been asleep for a while.

The facts are that rarely does the baby have conjunctivitis. Ninety-nine times out of hundred he does not have a contagious infection which can be passed to the other eye or to you. Secondly, the baby's sight will not be affected: what the baby has is a blocked tear duct.

If you look at the inner corner of your eye, you will able to see a fleshy bead-shaped structure. This is the tear sac, which collects the tears secreted by the eye, and passes them down a narrow tube (the tear duct) to the cavity of your

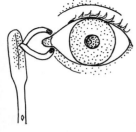

When a tear sac is blocked by a plug of mucus, the tear duct becomes infected, as shown in this cross-section.

nose. That's why your nose runs when you cry.

In babies there is a tendency for the bottom end of this duct to become blocked with a little plug of mucus. There is then a nice warm test tube of tears which incubates and grows whatever germs happen to be around at the time, and this produces the pus. The problem will disappear when the plug at the bottom of the tube is cleared by the body's normal processes, but until then it requires a little treatment. Pressing gently with the fingertip from inner corner of the eye to halfway down the side of the nose will squeeze out fluid and pus from both ends of the tear duct. Do this for three strokes three times a day. Then clean the eye, ideally with saline but cooled, boiled water will do. If the eye becomes very gummy it is often helpful to then instil some antibiotic eyedrops which can be prescribed by your doctor. This does not cure the condition but tends to cut down the number of germs within the tear duct and stops dried pus from making the mucus plug even more difficult for the body's normal mechanisms to remove.

The tear duct massage should be continued until the eye has been clear for a few days. It is unusual for the problem to last for more than a few days and if it does, the treatment is just the same. Only if the stickiness and weeping of the eye continue for nine months or more does probing of the duct by an ophthalmologist have to be considered. Even then, delaying the probing still longer usually results in the duct clearing itself spontaneously.

NAILS

INGROWING TOENAILS

Many babies are born with very short toenails, especially on the big toes. The nails are quite normal and grow out without problem. Occasionally, as the nails grow, the skin against the nail's leading edge becomes red and inflamed. All that is required is a little local antiseptic for a week or so. Even if the skin starts developing crusty granulations it still requires no further treatment. Only the most severe cases need antibiotics or referral to a surgeon.

A good time to cut fingernails is during feeds, when your baby is so busy that he tends to keep his hands still.

▼▼▼

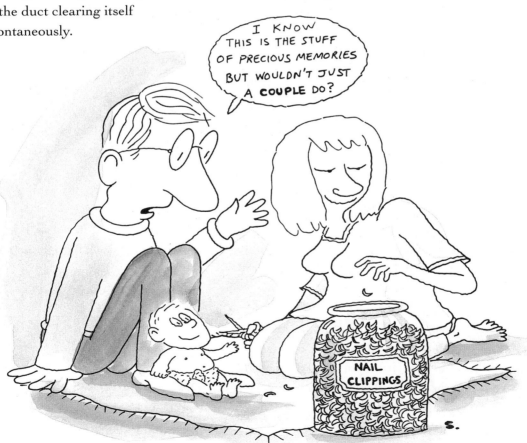

LONG FINGERNAILS

Full-term and post-term babies are frequently born with long fingernails. By coincidence, babies tend to hold their arms fully flexed at the elbow, which puts the sharp nails right up against the cheeks. Babies' cheeks are not meant to look lacerated so mothers usually want to cut the nails. For the first couple of weeks it is probably better to put cloth mittens on the hands to prevent this, rather than cut the nails. Attempting to trim soft, almost transparent, fingernails can be difficult — it is very easy to cut into the nail bed and draw blood. Later, although I do not advocate the mothercraft advice of biting your baby's nails, it is probably worthwhile to use clippers rather than scissors and go very carefully as it is easy to cut the nails too short. A good time to cut them is during feeds, when your baby is so busy that he tends to keep his hands still.

INFECTED NAILS

It is not unusual for the edges of the fingernails of babies to become red and inflamed after the first few days. The official name of the condition is paronychia. It usually starts where the corner of the nail meets the skin, often with a little of the cuticle flaking off. In the early stages local antiseptic is all that is required, but if the infection starts to spread towards the joint of the finger, then antibiotics are usually necessary.

SNUFFLES

Attention! This is an important sentence which will relieve much anxiety in the first days after the baby's birth: Don't worry, the baby does NOT have a cold.

Eight out of ten babies get fairly heavy snuffles in the first few days. The delicate lining of the nose produces lots of extra mucus to protect itself from an onslaught of milk and, if the baby regurgitates, acid gastric juice. When babies start to feed they are not particularly efficient about whether the milk goes down into the gullet or up into the nose. This is why the problem is so common. If the snuffles are interfering with the baby's sleeping or feeding, local decongestant or plain saline nasal drops can be helpful, but a word of warning: your baby will hate it. You will therefore be given a moving target and the nose is a pretty small target anyway.

My advice is to ignore the snuffles and they will go away.

COUGH

Occasionally, the amount of mucus produced by the nose can be so great that it pours out of the back of

Eight out of ten babies get fairly heavy snuffles in the first few days.
▼▼▼

the nose and down into the pharynx where it collects in the throat and gives the baby a 'rattly chest' or a cough. Again, this is usually nothing to worry about. If your baby really catches a cold or a viral infection he is likely to have not only snuffles or a cough but a raised temperature and will appear unwell. Also, the cough is more likely to then be repetitive and productive. You will know that he is just not himself, in which case hotfoot it to the doctor.

TOXIC ERYTHEMA

'THERE ARE FLEAS IN THIS HOSPITAL — AND THEY'RE BITING MY BABY.'

A day or so after delivery it is common for a baby to suddenly come out with a skin rash that makes him look as if he has been attacked by fleas or mosquitoes. The rash has a yellowish head with a surrounding wide red area. Occasionally there may be many such spots, which all run together making the baby look as if he has the measles. This rash is called 'toxic erythema' and is completely harmless and not the least toxic!

It seems to relate to the baby's skin first coming in contact with clothes, especially cotton. It does not mean the baby is allergic to anything or that he has particularly sensitive skin. The rash will go away after a few days and does not cause discomfort.

HICCUPS

You probably noticed your baby was hiccupping in the womb and now he hiccups outside. It tends to occur during or after feeds and these enormous hiccups rack his little body like convulsions! Don't worry. It is a sign of gratitude for a good feed and no treatment is necessary.

DRY SKIN

Most babies born at term, and all babies born post-term, develop dry skin in the days after delivery. At its most obvious, the skin can have deep cracks and fissures and the baby may slough off sheets of dead skin like a snake. More usually, though, the skin just gently scales and peels, especially over the hands and feet.

The top layer of skin that has been in contact with the amniotic fluid is merely being replaced and it doesn't mean the baby will have a permanently dry skin. It has no relationship to eczema and it needs no treatment.

However, moisturising with sorbolene, for example, will make the baby's skin look a little more like the proverbial baby's bottom!

Don't worry about hiccups. It's a sign of gratitude for a good feed. No treatment is necessary.

▼▼▼

Moisturising with sorbolene will make the baby's skin look a little more like the proverbial baby's bottom!

▼▼▼

PINK-STAINED NAPPIES

Sometimes mothers get a fright when they change their baby's nappy — the urine appears to be bloodstained! In fact, it is not blood but a pinkish-staining chemical called 'urate' which the babies pass in high concentration for the first few days after delivery. It is quite normal.

Little girls sometimes do have bloodstained nappies. A proportion of baby girls actually menstruate following the withdrawal of the hormones they had from the placenta. If they don't actually produce blood, most of them will produce a vaginal discharge in the first few days and this is quite normal. Many girls will also have a mucus tag hanging from the back of the vagina. This is also caused by stimulation from the hormones from the placenta and disappears after a few days or weeks.

Most newborns are 'double-jointed', and their hip joints have a fair amount of give between the ball and the socket. This is normal.

▼▼▼

GOOD URINARY STREAM

While we are on the subject of nappies, most little boys show their respect for their mother at an early stage by weeing over her. This shower offers you a chance to make a worthwhile observation! It means the baby's urinary stream is perfectly normal. If the urine just dribbles out of the little boy it is a good idea to let your paediatrician or midwife know. Occasionally such babies can have flaps in their urinary passage from the bladder, which prevent a good stream and can cause problems if left untreated. This problem does not occur in little girls.

CONGENITAL DISLOCATION OF HIPS

Babies are quite often born with a condition called 'clicky hips', and, far less commonly, with a congenital dislocation of the hip.

Many mothers have heard of 'clicky hips' but few have a clear idea what this means. Indeed, even doctors who study the subject closely are still in the dark about some aspects of this condition.

One of the many functions of the female hormones produced by the placenta is to soften the mother's ligaments to make the birth of the baby easier. These hormones cross the placenta and have a similar effect on the newborn baby. Consequently, most newborns are 'double-jointed' and their hip joints, which are ball-and-socket joints, have a fair amount of give between the ball and the

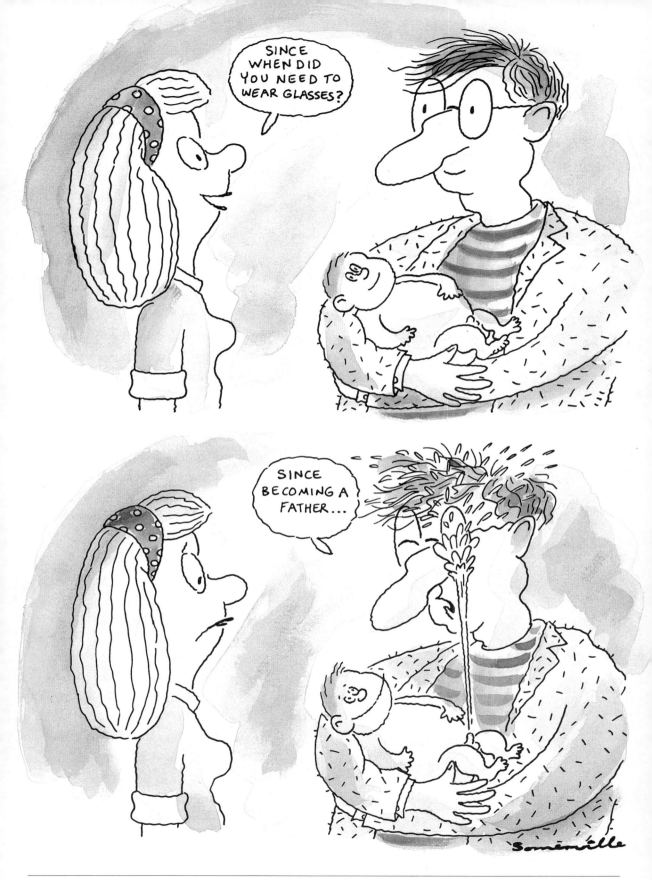

socket. This is, of course, a normal phenomenon. However, in some babies this looseness may represent not just lax ligaments but the possibility of developing an abnormally shallow socket.

It is most important that babies who will develop shallow sockets are discovered as early on in life as possible so that treatment to form a normally deep socket can be started. This condition, even at its worst, is curable, but only if we can spot these babies early on, preferably before the age of six months. We call the condition 'congenital dislocation of the hip' or CDH.

We know that, especially in girls, certain groups of babies are more likely to have this propensity. These are:

- those with a family history of congenital dislocation of the hip;
- breech births;
- babies who had only a small amount of amniotic fluid;
- babies who have other evidence of a cramped environment in the uterus;
- babies who are found to have clicky hips on examination following birth;
- first-born babies.

These factors are cumulative. For instance, if your baby is a girl, firstborn and a breech delivery, the chances of needing treatment

for CDH becomes as common as 1 in 15 babies.

The examination of the baby's hips should always be done by someone skilled at detecting CDH. It involves holding the hip firmly at right angles to the axis of the body with the baby on his back facing the examiner who then gently attempts to push the ball of the leg bone (femur) backwards out of the socket. Having done that, the leg is then rotated outwards so the baby is in a 'frog' posture. This tests the stability of the joint to dislocation.

If the head of the femur can be persuaded to leave the socket or there is excess 'give' in the joint, most paediatricians prescribe a 'Pavlik harness'. This is a device of straps and Velcro which holds the hips up at right angles to the axis of the body — not in the frog posture like some old-fashioned devices. All this one does is stop the baby stretching his legs out. He is free to move the knees apart or almost together.

This harness is a bit of a nuisance but that is all.

It is usually all right to bathe your baby a couple of times a week without the harness but the rest of the time the harness should be worn. Occasionally your doctor may not even allow removal during bathing — you should ask. After a short time, though, you'll all get used to it and usually it'll only be on for about 12 weeks. When it comes

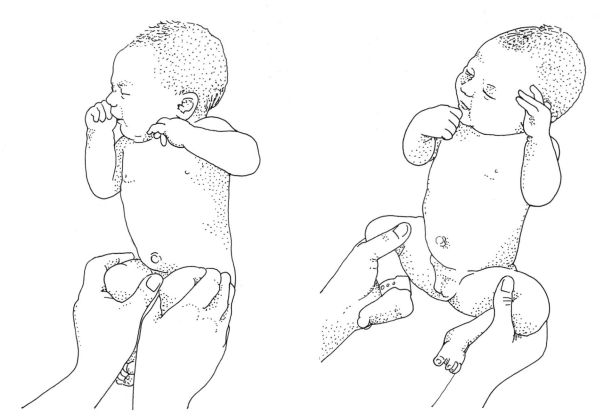

Left: The general posture of the newborn: arms and legs bent, head to the side, and trunk straight.
Right: The hip joints of all new babies are tested for signs of 'clicky hips'.

off, your baby's hips will be normal for the rest of his life — so it's worth it.

For all these babies, and any others in the high-risk groups, it is important to get a hip x-ray at the age of four to five months. Before this age the hip joint is made mostly of cartilage, not bone, so unfortunately the x-rays cannot show the joint properly. The x-ray will be able to exclude CDH, and though it is an unusual condition, it is critical that it is found no later than this age.

However, it has recently been found that ultrasound can be used at an earlier age, even in the new-born, and this test is getting more and more popular as its value is understood. Nevertheless, the x-ray remains the 'gold standard' for the diagnosis and should still be used as well.

In the first few months, there is another useful physical sign of the possibility of CDH. When the baby is lying on his back on the change table, normally the hips can be spread apart so that the knees can touch the surface of the table (or nearly). If it feels like there is a block to that movement, it is worth getting your paediatrician to examine your baby's hips, just to be on the safe side.

> *When the Pavlik harness comes off, your baby's hips will be normal for the rest of his life.*
>
> ▼▼▼

As a rule, babies should be dressed in the same number of layers and thickness of clothing as you are.

▼▼▼

Be very careful about exposing your baby to direct sunlight, especially within the first week of life.

▼▼▼

FEVERS

Many babies have a little fever on day two or day three and this does not represent infection or any problem. It usually coincides with the baby being at his driest, that is, after he has lost the extra water in his body and before the milk has come in.

At this age babies are very susceptible to overwrapping. So make sure, if the weather is warm, that he does not have too much covering him. As a rule, babies should be dressed in the same number of layers and thickness of clothing as you are. Babies do not need specially warm clothes unless conditions are very cool.

The problem with babies' temperature control is not that they need more insulation than older people but that they cannot compensate for rapid changes. If we are outside in thin clothes and a cold change comes through, our bodies compensate for that change by shivering and closing down our skin blood flow, retaining the warmth of the core of our bodies. Small babies are not able to compensate as efficiently, so care must be taken to dress the baby appropriately for the current environment, and if the temperature changes, respond accordingly.

Be very careful about exposing your baby to direct sunlight, especially within the first week of life. As their bodies are relatively fluid-deficient in this time, direct sunlight can cause a rapid rise in body temperature which can be very harmful. So avoid sun kicks until he is a few weeks older — even then it is wise to take special care.

WEIGHT LOSS

When babies are in the womb they are, in effect, marine animals, floating in a primordial sea. When they are born, their bodies are relatively waterlogged and they need to get rid of all that extra water. Nature has arranged this in a very clever way. Firstly, your milk does not come in for a couple of days so the baby does not drink very much. This allows him to get rid of his extra water. Secondly, he passes urine at a normal rate and therefore loses weight. This is absolutely normal. Many babies will lose up to 10 per cent of their body weight (that is 350 g or 12 oz in a normal-sized baby). And this is another reason babies are relatively uninterested in feeding in the first couple of days. Nature tells them that it's not necessary.

FAT NECROSIS

Some babies develop rubbery lumps under the skin after a few days, usually along the line of the jaw or the cheekbone. This is due to the fat cells in the skin rupturing during delivery. This releases fat into the tissue under the skin, which sets up an inflammatory reaction. It's quite harmless and the lumps will disappear in a few weeks.

DUMMIES AND THUMB-SUCKING

If a baby wants to suck, he should be allowed to do so. If you don't give him a dummy, he will probably find his fingers or his thumb. In fact a recent study showed that about a third of two-and-a-half-year-olds sucked fingers or thumbs and another third used dummies. All the bad reports about dummies are untrue. However, a 'dormel' (a miniature bottle filled with sugary drink) dissolves teeth and should never be used. The thumb is probably more convenient than the dummy and tends not to fall on the floor out of reach. Some parents reject dummies because of the appearance, others prefer their babies to have dummies because at some time in the future they can be thrown away (the dummies, that is!). The baby is sucking his thumb or dummy for very good reasons — it calms him, helps him sleep and comforts him. His parents' opinions of the aesthetic aspects don't interest him, and they should mind their own business.

Dummies don't cause disease,

If your baby wants to suck, he should be allowed to do so. The baby is sucking his thumb or dummy for very good reasons — it calms him, helps him sleep and comforts him.

▼▼▼

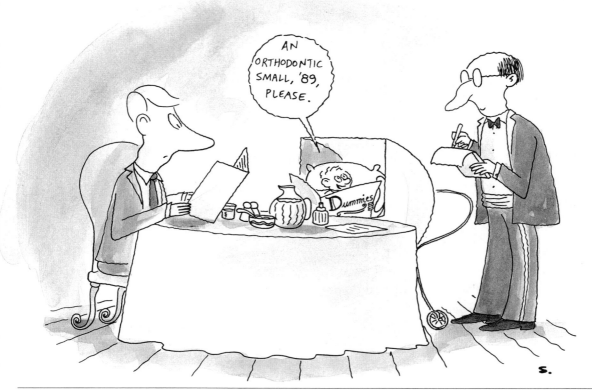

Dummies don't cause disease, and thumbs won't make his teeth stick out and cost you a fortune in orthodontics.

▼▼▼

and thumbs won't make his teeth stick out and cost you a fortune in orthodontics. Neither will his thumb shrink. For everyone's peace of mind, allow your baby to make up his mind about whether or not he wishes to suck and, if so, what.

SWEATING

It is not uncommon for babies to sweat profusely from their head, enough to wet the bedclothes. The cause is unknown but the sweating creates no problem and is not associated with any disease.

BLUE AROUND THE MOUTH

There is an amazing old wives' tale linking babies who have blue colouration around their mouth with colic. Don't ask me the connection because there is none. This colouration probably relates to congestion of the veins after a vigorous bout of sucking from the baby and is of no significance at all.

TONGUE-TIE

There is a thin membrane on the underside of the tongue in the midline which connects it to the floor of the mouth. This is a normal

structure. Occasionally it can extend far forward, nearly to the tip of the tongue. This is called tongue-tie. Rumours circulate that if the membrane extends far forward then it needs to be surgically incised. This information is incorrect. As the tongue grows, the membrane will retreat to its more normal position. While it still extends to the front of the tongue, it causes no problem with feeding, crying or anything else, for that matter. It should be left alone. Very rarely the membrane is thick and fleshy and indeed may restrict movement of the tongue to a degree that the young child (not baby) cannot lick his upper lip. Under these circumstances it might be necessary to get a surgical consultation, but not until the child is two years old.

UMBILICAL CLEANING

The umbilical cord is usually not the mother's favourite part of her baby. Most will touch it only reluctantly and fear that any handling will cause it to start bleeding or hurt the baby in some way.

The facts are that the cord has no pain fibres and cutting the cord didn't hurt the baby at all. Within an hour of delivery, the arteries are in spasm and bleeding is most unlikely. As long as the cord remains uninfected, important bleeding is impossible after the first day. Spots of blood from the cord are not a problem. The cord is very tough.

The cord should be cleaned at regular intervals because germs grow readily on its surface, and especially in the gutter between the cord and the skin. To clean it in hospital, use diluted methylated spirits, and while doing so, gently pull on the cord to get down into the gutter. If your baby cries while this is being done, it is not because it is painful but because the methylated spirits is cold to his skin. If the cord gets smelly, clean it more frequently. If the skin around the umbilicus becomes red, it may be developing an infection, so tell your paediatrician or midwife.

Once you get home you can stop using the spirits as there is then no danger of cross-infection. Just clean the cord with a dry cotton bud and it should fall off soon after. Cords can last between four days and six weeks.

FOURTH-DAY BLUES

The fourth day is a bitch. Your milk has just come in and you have these two beach balls on your chest. Your baby is slightly jaundiced and you don't know what is going on with him. He has been feeding two-hourly for the last 24 hours and you can't remember ever feeling so tired before. The newness and delight of the birth is starting to fade and you feel just plain depressed. Everyone who comes to see you looks only at the baby and tells you how wonderful you must be feeling. Your bottom is sore and you can't sit comfortably, or if you had a Caesarean, your incision hurts. On top of that, opening your bowels is difficult and very painful.

Many of the problems with the baby seem to explode out of all proportion today. He seems to have an insurmountable feeding problem. You suspect his jaundice is not the normal type but some new disease. When he cries, he seems to be blaming you for being born and you are sure all the doctors and nurses think you're a lot of trouble. The fact that your common sense tells you that all this is untrue is not much help. But these feelings will soon pass.

The only comforting thing to say about this picture of woe is that most mothers go through it. It seems to be related to the withdrawal of the high levels of placental hormones which were, believe it or not, putting you on a 'high' during your pregnancy. Day four seems to bring all these things to a head and my recommendation is to find a quiet corner (the shower

Fourth-day blues — when the newness and delight of the birth is starting to fade and you can't remember ever feeling so tired before.

▼▼▼

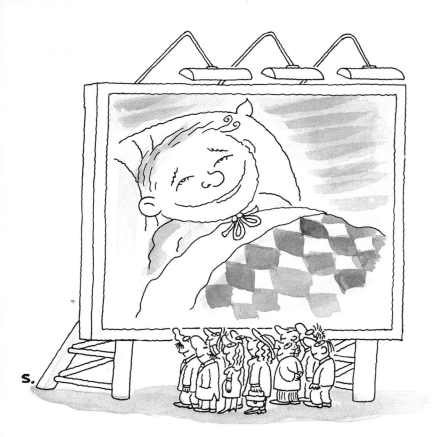

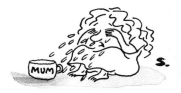

is a popular choice) and have a good cry.

Sometimes this depression can last several days or even longer, but that is unusual (see the chapter 'Postnatal Depression'). If it seems to be happening to you, do not keep it to yourself. It is important, will be taken seriously and it can be treated. It is also probably more common than women let on.

THE NEWBORN SCREENING TEST

The Newborn Screening Test is a blood test performed on your baby in the first week after birth. A blood sample is taken by a heel-prick and the blood absorbed onto a special piece of blotting paper. The sample is dried and sent to a central laboratory for testing. This screening test is designed to pick out those very few babies who have some rare diseases called 'inborn errors of metabolism'. That is, they are born missing some functions concerned with the breakdown of food into the building blocks of the body and/or the building up of body tissues from those building blocks. These disorders are extremely rare (1 in 30,000 to 100,000).

The Newborn Screening Test these days incorporates two other important tests. One tests the thyroid function and will pick up if your baby's thyroid is not producing enough hormone (this is an important cause of brain damage if it is not picked up immediately). The other tests for cystic fibrosis. This is a disease of the excreting glands of the body which has important effects in the baby's lungs and digestive system.

You are not informed of a negative result of these tests. However, it is not unusual for the laboratory to ask for a further sample in the case of a borderline result or laboratory problems. Under these circumstances, the test will almost always be negative and the laboratory will inform you of this result as soon as the test is done.

If the test happens to be positive you will hear about it soon after the test is done.

JAUNDICE

Usually on the second or third day most babies' skin starts to go a little yellow in colour. This is jaundice. As the days go on this colour may deepen and cause the whites of the eyes to become yellow also.

This jaundice of infancy has no relationship to the jaundice in older children and adults, which is associated with illnesses, especially of the liver. The baby's jaundice is just part of the normal process of the baby adapting to life outside his mother's womb.

THE CAUSE

Jaundice is caused by a substance called bilirubin, which is the breakdown product of haemoglobin, the red pigment in blood. Every day 1 per cent of the red blood cells in the body is being broken down, and this produces bilirubin. While the baby is in the womb this bilirubin is passed across the placenta and processed by the mother's liver so that it can be excreted. The fetus's liver needs to do very little of this work. Once the baby has been born, however, his liver has to 'learn' how to process the bilirubin for itself. This takes a few days, and up until that time the jaundice level of the baby will rise steadily. In most babies it never rises to a high level and nothing need be done about it.

However, in some babies the level may continue to rise higher than average. In VERY high quantities, circulating bilirubin can be dangerous to a baby. It is therefore a good idea to make sure that the jaundice reaches nowhere near such levels. Your doctor can estimate the jaundice level of the baby by pressing his nose and observing the colour of the skin and noting how far the jaundice colour extends down his body. Some hospitals nowadays are a bit more sophisticated and monitor the level using devices that flash a standard dose of light against the baby's skin.

Jaundice of infancy has no relationship to the jaundice in older children and adults, which is associated with illnesses.
▼▼▼

Jaundice is just part of the normal process of the baby adapting to life outside his mother's womb.
▼▼▼

The jaundice pigment in the skin absorbs the blue colour in the light and the device measures the amount of light absorbed to estimate the level of jaundice. If these screening levels appear higher than average, the bilirubin level will be measured and followed, using blood tests, once or twice a day. In addition, other blood tests may be ordered to check for other conditions that increase the rate of red blood cell breakdown in the body, such as incompatibility between the baby's and the mother's blood groups.

If the level is found to be rising quickly, or rising to moderate levels, your doctor will start treatment. It must be emphasised, however, that the safety margin is very large and while the baby is under such care, there is no danger to his health.

PHOTOTHERAPY

The level of jaundice in the baby can be controlled using phototherapy. This is a simple procedure, where the naked baby is exposed to ordinary fluorescent light. The bilirubin absorbs the energy from the light and this energy breaks the bilirubin down so that it can be easily excreted. We use the phototherapy as a holding measure until the baby's liver is able to handle the bilirubin for itself.

While the baby is under phototherapy, pads are put over his eyes to stop him being dazzled and help him sleep. These pads do have a tendency to slip off and they should be gently replaced.

When the baby first goes under the lights, his temperature will be taken occasionally to make sure that he doesn't get cold. He is fed as normal. Some jaundiced babies, however, are a bit sleepy and are rather lazy on the breast. Under these circumstances, it may be advisable to express your milk and give it to the baby in a bottle, or (but this unusual) to give the baby some formula if feeding is not established. Once the baby's jaundice level starts to come down he usually wakes promptly and feeds much better, so this becomes just another holding procedure and does not mean that the bottle needs to be continued.

As the jaundice is broken down by the light, the breakdown products are passed out in the stool. These tend to make the stool rather more loose and frequent than before. Also, you may notice it becomes more greenish in colour. These changes merely demonstrate that the phototherapy is doing its job and the jaundice is being eliminated from the body.

Occasionally some babies (not being used to sunbathing) tend to cry for the first few hours under the lights. This phase will quickly pass as the baby adjusts to his new circumstances.

PROLONGED JAUNDICE

The jaundice level starts to come down from about day five onwards, with or without the lights. It then usually drops rapidly over the next few days and, unless it looks like it's increasing (a rare happening), it should be ignored. However, it is not unusual for the jaundice, though paler, to remain for some weeks and you can get pretty sick of your friends commenting on your lemon-yellow baby!

Such babies are almost invariably breastfed. It seems that some substance in the milk stops the baby's liver completely eliminating the jaundice. It never does any harm at all and if you wait it will slowly fade and disappear. If you're tired of your friends' amusing references to the little lemon, you could try stopping breastfeeding for 48 hours. During this time, feed the baby formula and express your breasts to keep up your milk flow. (Freeze the milk for the baby-sitter to use later.) This might hasten the disappearance of the jaundice but it doesn't always work.

NAMING THE BABY

After a few years in this game I now realise that there is no way I ought to write this section. Naming babies is a deeply personal process and often bears little relationship to logic, aesthetics, common sense or foresight. People can get very fond of the weirdest names and I have now learned not to throw back my head and roar with laughter when I am told that a baby is going to be called Crudidge or Waffinberry. However, against my better judgment, I would like to impart a few little rules that have come my way:

- Remember your baby has to live with this name for the rest of his or her life. Within a short time he will even start to look like his name. So give him a name to be proud of, not to please a rich aunt, or to follow a family tradition, or because your favourite football team won the cup.
- If you give his name a strange spelling, he will have a lifetime of spelling it out for others. I think it is a real problem to use a common name with an uncommon spelling. So if you want to call your daughter Alison, don't spell it Allysoine.
- Cadence and rhythm are very important. Try the name out with the surname and see that it is easy to say and has a nice sound. Dalton Hilton just doesn't work.
- Be careful of initials. Avoid WC, VD, STD (think of all the telephone jokes...), BUM, and, more subtly, even RC.
- Humour is okay, but make sure the joke is going to last more than

Naming babies often bears little relationship to logic, aesthetics, commonsense or foresight.

a few months. I once had as a patient a 700 g (25 oz) premature baby whom the parents called Goliath for a laugh. I don't know if this little lad appreciated it when he was 14 years old.

- Try to avoid fashion. Some babies who were born in the 1960s are probably now pretty sick of their names, especially Freelove Jones or Moonglow Smith. Also, if you're the fifteenth John in your class at school it can be a pain, so check the papers for the latest common names and avoid them.
- Some people have to use family names. However, why not make that their second name and make their first name a nice one?
- Don't feel pressured to name your baby in the first few days. If you need the time, take it. Also, don't feel embarrassed about changing your mind a few days (or weeks) down the road. It's an important issue.

An obstetrics friend of mine has a great system that he recommends. The parents go into separate rooms and write a list of their ten favorite names, scoring each one out of ten in preference order. They then swap lists and delete all those names they hate. The others are then scored out of ten. It is usual that there are a couple of names that both give scores over seven or eight and they can work on them without wasting time on names that

have no chance of getting up with the partner. In the event of a tie they toss for it or fight!

FROM PARTNER TO FATHER

It cannot be a coincidence that so many diverse cultures exclude fathers from the birth process. It is as if they fear that the father might get too involved in his newborn baby and neglect his role as provider. It just would not do for dad to spend all day playing with his baby by the hearth when there is no food in the pantry. Studies of fathers' response to their newborns seem to validate this conclusion. If they were very involved in the birth process, most fathers exhibit much the same behaviour as mothers when presented with their babies — some taking quite a dominant role in handling and playing with the baby. Certainly, they seemed totally engrossed with the little one and positively bursting with self-esteem. You can usually recognize a new dad: he's the one with terminal fatigue in his smiling muscles.

It must be said that a father cannot be as involved with his baby as a breastfeeding mother. Babies tend to treat their fathers with indifference for a few weeks, as they are mostly interested in the smell, taste and milk of their mother. Most fathers can handle this without getting upset or jealous but it is a good idea to involve the father as much as possible in all the caretaking activities he can do. Literally, the more he does for the baby, the closer he will feel to him. This is one of the few advantages of bottle-feeding, allowing the parenting role to be divided more equally between mother and father.

SUPERDAD

Some early studies on bonding assessed the closeness of the relationship between mother and baby, using a description of the way the mother behaved while the doctor examined her baby. If she stood on the other side of the room gazing out of the window, and when the baby cried, turned around and muttered, 'Oh, he's always doing that', she scored a big zero. If she stood next to the doctor and immediately pacified him when he cried (the baby, that is — doctors are pretty brave), she scored a six.

I recently had a big burly dockside worker and his wife in my consulting room, for their baby's checkup. The mother had been quite sick and had to remain in

You can usually recognize a new dad: he's the one with terminal fatigue in his smiling muscles.

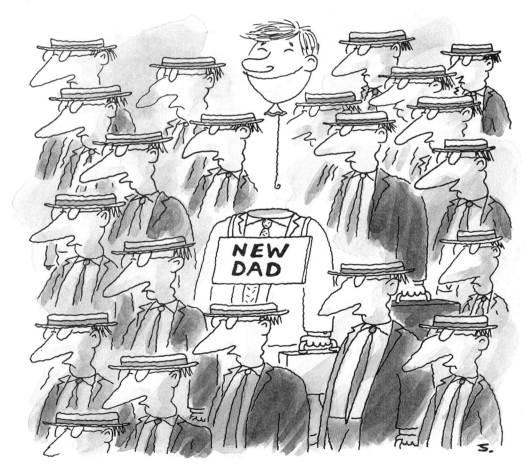

The more dad
does for the
baby, the
closer he will
feel to him.

▼▼▼

hospital for four weeks following the birth of her baby. Hence the husband had looked after all the baby's needs and had bottle-fed him. When I examined the baby, I had to contend with an enormous shoulder in my way, as father got a score of seven out of six for bonding!

FATHERS GET ATTACHED TOO

As a young neonatologist in the Newborn Transport Team, I once flew 480 km (300 miles) from Denver to a small town in Kansas, in the USA. We were to pick up a baby girl who had become sick within the first few days after birth.

At the hospital I met the parents and reassured them that we would stabilise her and then fly her back to Denver Children's Hospital in our aircraft. The little girl required an hour or so of stabilisation before we took off. As we wheeled the little girl in through the doors of the Denver Hospital, the father was there to greet us. He had beaten our flight to Denver in his car (and had received only one speeding ticket!). He watched over her cot until she was out of danger.

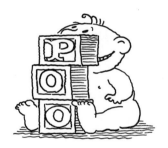

CHAPTER 4

BREAST IS BEST

It's cheap, easily transportable,
doesn't need sterilising and it's perfect
for the baby in every way.

Breast is best! There's no argument about it. It's cheap, easily transportable, doesn't need sterilising and it's perfect for the baby in every way. Breastfeeding virtually immunises him against bacterial gastroenteritis and there is a lower incidence of respiratory tract and middle ear infections in breastfed babies.

Breast milk is always readily available at the right temperature, and best of all, breastfeeding is enjoyable. Having your baby sucking on your breast can release wonderful pleasure-producing hormones which tranquillise and reward you for doing it.

However, it is much better if you want to breastfeed your baby for reasons other than because you think it's good for him. Self-sacrifice is something all children expect from their mother, but not in this instance. Babies prefer their mother to feed them in the way that makes her happier, more relaxed and less tired. If breastfeeding does that, and for most

it will, go for it; but if you feel that the bottle is the way to go for you, go for that.

Getting started with breastfeeding is not necessarily easy. It is a strange phenomenon: in primates (that is, higher mammals such as apes) breastfeeding is not an instinctive ability, so it needs to be taught. In chimpanzee troupes in the wild the older females teach the younger ones how to do it. Zoo experience with gorillas has taught us the same thing. Because there are usually only a few in any zoo, if a gorilla has a baby there is usually no experienced female to teach her how to feed the little one. To overcome this, techniques such as allowing the gorilla to watch humans breastfeed, or videotapes of gorillas feeding their young, have been used. Unfortunately this has often had only limited success.

Maternity hospitals have lots of experienced staff to help you get started — make sure you make use of this vital resource.

*Make sure
you are both
comfortable
and relaxed.*

▼ ▼ ▼

ATTACHING THE BABY TO THE BREAST

Many babies, if allowed to do so, will suck on the nipple like a bottle teat. This is the wrong technique, producing no colostrum for him and soreness (and even blistering) of the nipple for you. Getting your baby attached properly is critical to breastfeeding, so get the best help you can for the early feeds.

Your baby should be presented with the breast before he is howling and tense, ideally, so you and he are as relaxed as possible. Make sure you are comfortable, sitting or lying on your side. Unwrap the baby so that you can both enjoy the skin contact — if it's a cool day put a blanket over both of you. Gently talk to him and let his lips stroke your nipple. He should respond by opening his mouth wide and 'rooting' for it. The idea then is to

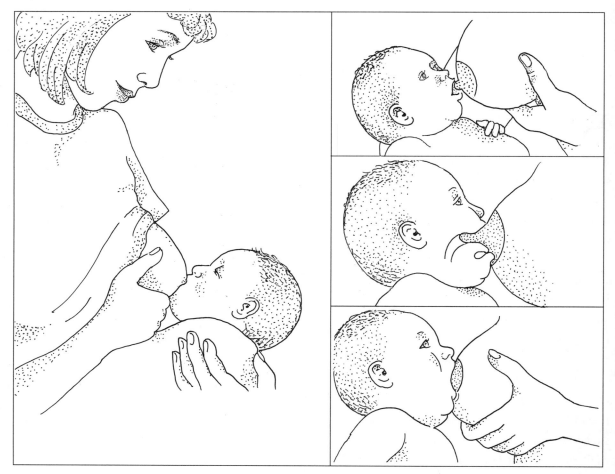

For successful breastfeeding, a comfortable position is essential. Let the baby's lips stroke the nipple, and he should respond by opening his mouth and 'rooting' for it. The cross-section shows the slightly upward position of the nipple in the baby's mouth, and the position of his tongue and gums. The nipple is immobilised by suction against the palate, while the jaws chomp and the tongue rolls from the front to the back of the mouth.

get the whole of the nipple into his mouth so he can hold it by suction up against the back of his palate. This will draw much of the areola (the pigmented area around the nipple) into his mouth, so that there may be only a rim of it outside his mouth above and none below. This immobilises the breast and allows him to squeeze the milk ducts which lie under the areola. He does this by:

• chomping on that area with jaw action. You can see the muscles right out to his ears move as he does it. If he sucks in his cheeks, he's not on properly;

• a rolling action with his tongue, from the front of his mouth to the back.

Once the flow has started and there is an unbroken column of milk down his throat, the milk will 'siphon' out of the breast.

Both of these actions cause the colostrum or milk to squirt out of the breast into his throat to be swallowed. The process usually has some help from the 'let-down' reflex.

The nipple is only used to immobilise the breast in the mouth. There is no rubbing of the skin and no reason for soreness to develop if the attachment is right.

THE LET-DOWN REFLEX

The ducts that collect the milk produced in the milk sacs of the breast lie deep in the breast. They have muscle fibres in their walls, and under the action of the hormone oxytocin (the same hormone that contracts your uterus), they contract and eject their milk. This explains the afterpains you get in your uterus, especially when you feed the baby, and why feeding the baby soon after delivery is so good to help the uterus contract.

In the early days the let-down is often not felt but can be detected as a change in the suck/swallow rhythm of the baby as a surge of milk enters his mouth. It also may produce a sudden thirst in the mother, so having a glass of water at hand during a feed is a good routine.

After a few weeks, when the breast is less engorged, a mother can often feel this reflex as a tingle at the beginning of a feed. Sometimes a hungry cry from her baby is enough on its own to initiate the let-down reflex.

SEVEN STEPS TO SUCCESSFUL BREASTFEEDING

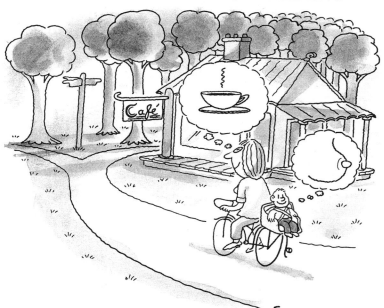

1 Start as early as possible, hopefully in the first couple of hours and certainly within the first twelve.

2 Make sure an experienced midwife teaches you how to attach your baby to the breast properly from the beginning.

3 Demand feed the baby right from the start. Give him unlimited access.

4 Feed the baby for as long as he wants to at every feed — within reason. If the feeds are taking longer than 30 minutes after the milk has come in, perhaps he's not attached well or his positioning is wrong so he finds it difficult to swallow.

5 If your nipples get sore, it's a warning that something needs adjusting, either the baby's attachment to the breast or his position. It's not that he's sucking too long or that he's sucking too vigorously.

6 Don't miss the night feeds. It's likely they boost your milk supply even more than daytime feeds. Feeding is also tranquillising and may help you sleep better.

7 Don't wash your nipples other than in normal hygiene. The nipple produces substances that attract your baby and help him attach to the breast. Don't use creams, lotions, potions or that magic ointment that the old lady round the corner says will stop nipple soreness. Change breast pads often and try to spend a little time with your breasts uncovered. Studies show that the best thing for your nipples, sore or otherwise, is nothing at all.

POSITIONING THE BABY

- Make sure you are both comfortable and relaxed.
- Let the breast fall into the baby's mouth, don't put it there.
- The baby's head shouldn't be too flexed or extended — you try swallowing with your neck stretched or scrunched up!
- If you are having to press the breast to avoid it obstructing his nose, change his position so the nipple points more towards the roof of his mouth.
- The baby's body should face yours so that you're chest to chest.
- Supporting the baby on your arm with his body across the front of yours, or under your arm, are common positions. So is lying down with both of you on your side.

THE FIRST FEW DAYS

Many babies in the first two or three days are sleepy and not wildly enthusiastic about feeding. It's not really surprising as there is no more than a dribble of colostrum for them when they wake, and being sensible people, babies do only what is rewarding. Take the opportunity to get some rest because when your milk comes in, a little light will come on in your baby's head and your life will not be the same again!

COLOSTRUM

Sometimes even before you have had your baby, but in increasing quantities after, the breast produces colostrum. This is a clear to yellow-coloured fluid which is full of antibodies and immunity-promoting cells. These substances line the baby's bowel and set up the start of immunity against gastroenteritis. It is certainly good for the baby, but it is not too much of a problem if the baby misses out on it for any reason. The bowel will catch up when the breast milk is available.

MILK 'COMING IN'

The milk 'comes in' at about two-and-a-half days, and following that, especially for the next 24 hours, the baby demands to be fed much more often, sometimes every one or two hours. This can really wear you out, but have no fear. Your baby will settle down as he gets used to the milk and he will feed for longer periods of time, less frequently.

HOW LONG SHOULD FEEDING MY BABY TAKE?

You should feed your baby for as long as he likes, as long as it is less than about half an hour, unless you don't mind being used for comfort

Take the opportunity to get some rest in the first few days because when your milk comes in your life will not be the same again.

▼▼▼

The more the breast is emptied of milk and the more the breast is suckled, the more milk there will be produced.

▾▾▾

sucking and you both enjoy it. Ideally he should stay on the first breast until he stops sucking and falls off. It is not necessary to time him so he gets both breasts equally each feed. Actually towards the end of a feed the milk is richer in fat (hence relatively more calories) so he finds it more satisfying.

Indeed it seems that it is the total amount of fat that he gets from the feed that switches off his appetite at the end, not the feeling of stomach fullness. Of course if he wants more, then offer the other breast, but if he's not interested, don't. Then next feed, start with the other breast to even things up.

NOT ENOUGH MILK

The more the breast is emptied of milk and the more the breast is suckled, the more milk will be produced. It is a very neat feedback mechanism (no pun intended!). As for substances you can take to increase your milk flow (called lactogogues), other than a drug called Metaclopramide which has a small effect in some mothers and no effect in others, no-one has ever shown that anything makes any difference — not stout, brewer's yeast, herbs or extra fluids. So don't waste the time you could spend resting. If there were some effective

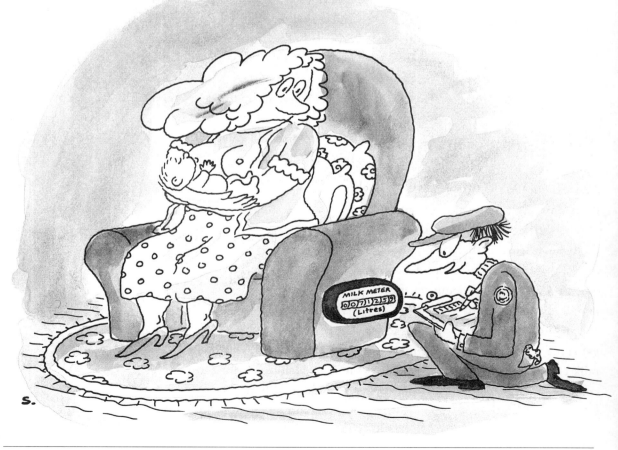

lactogogues available you can be sure that the dairy farmers would know about it — and they have no magic answers either.

In summary then, the three things that increase your milk supply are good breast emptying (the most important factor), more suckling at the breast and more rest for mother. And that's it.

WATER FEEDS

It is most unusual for your baby to become dehydrated, so he should not be offered water feeds. There is never a need for glucose and water as this will just make your baby vomit and will offer him very little nourishment. Your baby is very well designed to cope with barely a dribble of feed for two or three days or even longer so he will come to no harm if you both patiently await the arrival of breast milk.

TOO MUCH MILK

When the milk first comes in, very commonly the breasts become engorged — it could be called the 'beach ball syndrome'. Luckily this only lasts 12 to 24 hours and is usually relieved by cold packs, a couple of paracetamol tablets and gentle expression of a little of the milk to take the tension out of the breast. If the breasts are very tight,

the baby sometimes cannot attach properly and a little hand expression of milk before the feed can help soften them. Do not attempt to empty the breast as it will merely fill up again. Do not use mechanical milk expressers, only the hand ones. Also at this time (and thereafter while you are breastfeeding) use the best supporting bra you can find: nothing skimpy or necessarily attractive, but with thick straps and large enough cups so all of the breast is contained. Avoid tight bands across the tops of the breasts, which only encourage duct obstruction and mastitis.

SORE NIPPLES

Luckily the nipples have a very high blood flow, and if the attachment to the breast is corrected (sorry to go on about this so much but you're probably getting the message that it is crucial), they will heal rapidly. If you have a cracked or blistered nipple it is a good idea to gently express that breast and feed the baby only on the other side. Then start again on that breast after 24 hours. Only in extreme cases is gentle hand expression and feeding the baby breast milk from a bottle necessary. Nipples heal quickly, so hang in there.

Sometimes, at the start, breastfeeding can seem more trouble and pain than it's worth.

▼▼▼

THINGS NOT GOING WELL

Sometimes, at the start, breastfeeding can seem more trouble and pain than it's worth. The pain from a breast or nipple can be exquisite. This is not surprising, as it is such a sensitive organ even when it's not cracked or chewed and chomped on every couple of hours. A useful piece of advice, though: don't give up breastfeeding at 2 am.

In the middle of the night, when things have been going badly for some days, you're tired and weepy, the baby's hungry and howling, and you dread every feed because of the pain from your breasts, it's so easy just to chuck it all in and order the formula. In the morning, though, things often look different and you may regret your decision... but then you don't want to backtrack...

Hang in there till morning and make a clear-headed decision in the light of day. Even if it's the same decision, you'll feel better about how you made it.

By the way, if you change your mind you can still get your milk back some days after quitting.

HOW OFTEN SHOULD HE FEED?

If we look at other mammalian milks in the animal kingdom, we find that there is a relationship between the amount of fat in the milk and the interval between feeds. The whale feeds her baby once every 24 hours and the milk is thick and creamy. The deer has an eight-hourly milk, the dog, four-hourly. Contrary to what you may have been told, human milk is definitely not a four-hourly one. In fact, our milk is relatively diluted and seems to look like one (brace yourself!) that should be fed almost continually.

If we look at breastfeeding mothers in hunter-gatherer societies, we find that they feed their babies about every 15 minutes round the clock. Even at night the babies sleep with their mothers and are on and off the breast while the mother sleeps.

This probably represents the 'normal' human pattern and certainly it is this pattern that allows the contraceptive function of breastfeeding to work very efficiently. This is not because the baby is in the way, either, but through hormones secreted by the mother's pituitary in response to frequent suckling on her breast!

Our babies grow to be more reasonable in their demands as the days go on, purely as a cultural phenomenon in our society. They do what's expected of them. Some, however, take longer to space their feeds than others and cannot be pushed too soon. Whether your baby is a frequent snacker or a regular-as-clockwork gorger is just luck.

Remember, however, that the breast fills in about 30 minutes and a full baby's stomach takes about 50 minutes to empty so he's not being unreasonable if he wants to feed hourly. It usually doesn't take too long before the interval becomes longer.

So let your baby drive — he knows the way he wants to go and trying to manipulate his feed times might just make him worse.

LACTOSE INTOLERANCE

Lactose intolerance in the baby who has not suffered a bout of gastroenteritis is most unusual. It is normal for a fully breastfed baby to spill some lactose in his stool. These babies tend to be the ones who produce rather explosive frothy stools fairly frequently. This is not an indication to stop breastfeeding and it will usually pass with time. If, however, your baby is taking a few very large feeds, say four per day, you could attempt to feed him more

often. This may give the intestine the lactose more gradually and improve absorption. If, however, he tends to 'snack' and only takes the foremilk from the breasts, which contains mostly lactose but not much fat (and it's the fat that gives him satisfaction), he might be persuaded to feed for longer on the same breast to get the fat-rich hindmilk and therefore take less total volume of feed.

In extreme cases of lactose spillage into the stool, a few days on a lactose-free formula is usually enough to correct the situation and then breastfeeding should be reintroduced. But I emphasise, this situation is very unusual.

BURPING

Babies are better burpers than we are. The valve between the stomach and the gullet is extremely inefficient in newborn babies and develops better tone as the months pass. Many babies have a very poor hold on their feed and are very likely to posset or regurgitate parts of it during or after the feed. This is even more likely to occur if the baby is postured head down. Consequently, the idea that a baby can trap an air bubble behind this valve, which needs ritualised back-pounding to release it, doesn't make a lot of sense. If babies don't burp after they have been fed there are

If babies don't burp after they have been fed there are two possibilities: the baby didn't swallow any air and there is nothing to burp up or he will burp it up later.

Most babies vomit and rarely is this a sign of sickness.

BREASTFEEDING — BEWARE!

These drugs can be secreted in the milk in amounts that affect the baby.

- Tetracycline
- Anticancer drugs (antimetabolites or cytotoxics)
- Long-acting radioisotopes (if you have special x-ray examinations tell the doctor you're breastfeeding)
- Antithyroid drugs and iodides
- Bromide
- Oral hypoglycaemic agents (for diabetes)
- Some sex hormones (don't take higher dose oral contraceptives)
- Some cortisones (but prednisone is OK)
- Some antirheumatism drugs (gold salts, indomethacin or phenylbutazone)
- Antimigraine drugs containing ergot
- Heroin

DRUGS IN BREAST MILK

Most mothers who are on medication are very concerned that the drug might be passed through to the baby in the breast milk. Happily there are very few drugs which get into breast milk in quantities that have any effect on the baby.

All these are harmless:

- most common antibiotics
- anti-histamines
- antidepressants (even lithium)
- antihypertensives
- tranquillisers
- analgesics (aspirin, paracetamol, codeine)
- laxatives
- drugs that act on the heart.

If you are taking **anticonvulsants,** such as phenobarbitone or phenytoin, you can still breastfeed, but your doctor will make sure that the dosage is correct for you both.

The list would not be complete, however, if we left off **alcohol**, which is fine as long as you don't overdose, and **nicotine** from cigarette smoke, which isn't fine at all. In fact, one of the breakdown products of nicotine is found in large quantities in the milk and in the urine of babies of smoking mothers. Smoking has been implicated in increasing the incidence of cot death, childhood leukaemia, respiratory tract infections in the under-fives and reducing intelligence quotients in smokers' children. Some of this data is uncertain but who wants to take the risk? Do your little newcomer and yourself a big favour and quit.

If you are prescribed any drug you should, of course, tell the doctor you are breastfeeding, just to be on the safe side.

two possibilities: the baby didn't swallow any air and there is nothing to burp or he will burp it later.

Neither of these possibilities is to be feared. Air bubbles in the bowel do not cause pain or discomfort, distension or spasm. Following a feed, all you need to do is to sit the baby up and give him a cuddle and if he wishes to burp, he will. Can you imagine having a satisfying, filling, tranquillising, delightful meal, and then have someone pound you between the shoulder blades before the coffee? Better to let the baby drift off to sleep and put him gently back in his cot (for more on this see the chapter 'Colic and the Crying Baby').

VOMITING

The valve between the gullet and the stomach in the newborn baby is extremely weak. If this valve is hanging open as the stomach squeezes to push the milk down into the bowel, the milk is just as likely to be squeezed up and out. This vomiting can even be projectile. X-ray studies of newborn babies show that this possibility occurs in most babies, but it improves rapidly with time. If it occurs often enough to be a worry:

• Sit the baby up after feeds;
• Put him on his right side in his cot in a head-up position. Up to

30 degrees is ideal, but he will tend to slide down the cot unless you put him in a carrying harness with the straps tied to the top of the cot.

Often after vomiting the baby will need topping up right away.

What a pity it is that we use the expression 'being sick' for vomiting. Most babies vomit and rarely is this a sign of sickness.

TWINS AND MORE

Twins are rather more than twice the work of one. Under these circumstances forget ideology. If one is awake and hungry, wake the other baby and feed them both — either together (the easier method if you've got the technique of attaching one to each breast) or one straight after the other.

Demand feeding is usually too hard and you'll be dead on your feet in a week. Some mothers can feed both babies entirely on the breast and it is definitely worth a try. However, it's a lot of milk to produce, especially in the face of tiredness, so keep an eye on their weight gain and complement with formula if necessary.

Do your little newcomer and yourself a big favour: quit smoking.

▼▼▼

Babies will provide themselves with the right amount of calories if offered the breast and allowed to direct when to stop and when to switch breasts.

▼▼▼

IN SUMMARY

Except for the technique of attachment and positioning, your baby needs very little supervision regarding his feeding. Nature is not so dumb that you need three hands, a stopwatch, electronic scales and tubes of nipple cream in order to successfully feed your baby. The correct phrase to describe the process is 'baby-led' feeding. We know from detailed research that babies will provide themselves with the right amount of calories if offered the breast (and often only one is necessary) and allowed to direct when to stop and when to switch breasts.

DOING BOTH

It is usually fairly difficult to both breast- and bottle-feed except as a temporary measure, for instance when weaning the baby off the breast or trying to build up one's milk supply. Doing both, you get many of the disadvantages of both methods and few of the advantages of either. Formula dilutes the antibodies in breast milk that protect the baby from bacterial gastroenteritis, and the convenience of bottle-feeding is lost if you also have to breastfeed. Feeding can also take too long. However, there may be some subtle advantages to any amount of breast milk, such as tiny amounts of growth factors, hormones and other substances only half-understood at present. So do both if it suits you both.

BOTTLE-FEEDING

If you want to bottle-feed your baby, do so. The main advantage of breastfeeding is that it is easier. If that is not the case in your life, then don't let anybody make you feel guilty about it. Babies prefer their mothers to be well rested and happy. An advantage of bottle-feeding is that dad and other people can help out, which, particularly if you are a working mother, is very helpful.

The formulas available today are nutritionally very similar to breast milk, and using them, babies will thrive and grow at just the same rate. They are derived from cow's milk or use vegetable protein from the soya bean. There are many different formulas available and all are now 'humanised', meaning they contain close to the same amount of protein, carbohydrate, fat and minerals as breast milk. In addition, many also contain extra vitamins and iron in recommended dosages. In choosing a formula, get the one that is easiest for you to obtain and stick to it. Don't listen too hard to other mothers' stories or you'll be chopping and changing every time junior vomits. None of the major formulas make babies vomit (but they all taste awful to adults). Most of them are available in concentrated liquid or powdered form, the former being marginally easier to make up, but rather more expensive.

Using formula, it is very important to observe cleanliness of hands and sterility of bottle and teat. Set aside a can-opener and knife (for smoothing off the scoops of powder) just for making up the formula and prepare a whole 24 hours' supply in one go, keeping the made-up formula in the refrigerator. Make up rather more than you calculate he actually needs for the day. Boil the water for the formula for a full ten minutes, then let it become lukewarm before pouring it into a sterile jug (or his bottle) and adding level scoops of formula powder. Never add any more powder than is recommended in the directions on the tin, as the exact concentration of powder in the water is critical.

An advantage with bottle-feeding is that dad and other people can help out.

▼▼▼

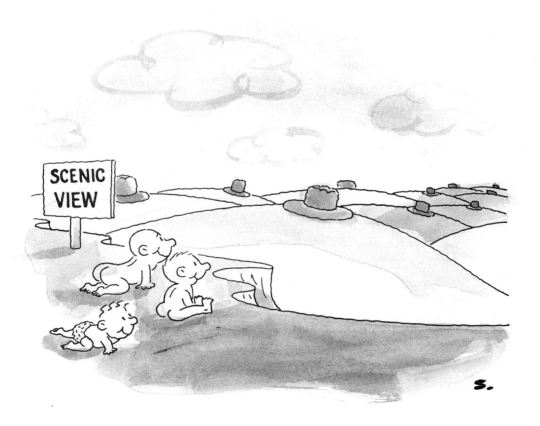

He should be demand fed — when he's hungry, not by the clock. At the end of the feed if there is something left in the bottle and he's not sucking anymore, he's had enough.

▼▼▼

When you feed him his bottle, treat it as you would a breastfeed. Give him all your attention and, if you like, your skin contact. He would enjoy it if you took your blouse off and cuddled him during a feed, and you probably would too. You needn't actually warm his formula because babies will take their milk cold just as well, but that's up to you.

How much you feed him is up to him. He should be demand fed when he's hungry, not fed by the clock. At the end of the feed if there is something left in the bottle and he's not sucking anymore, he's had enough.

On average (note the emphasis) a baby takes about 160 ml per kilogram (or about 3 fl oz per pound) of his body weight a day, but that's an average baby on an average day. Don't insist on exact amounts each feed. Like us, sometimes he'll want more and sometimes less.

When he's finished, rinse the bottle and teat straight away to remove formula before it dries, and always discard formula left over in the bottle from a feed or at the end of 24 hours.

Beware of using microwave ovens for warming formula or for thawing frozen breast milk. They really heat the milk but the bottle still feels cold. Anyway, always check the temperature of the milk by sprinkling a little from the bottle onto the inner part of your wrist.

Remember, if you are travelling to a developing country, be very careful of bad water supply or drainage and make sure reliable refrigeration is available. Your baby is vulnerable to gastroenteritis if he is bottle-fed. Under these circumstances a real effort to breastfeed is very worthwhile.

CHAPTER 5

POSTNATAL DEPRESSION

*Postnatal depression is a catch-all phrase
covering severe depressive mood change.
It is most important to admit the problem
and talk to someone who understands. .*

You've seen the advertisements. A beautiful woman, looking as if her day job is modelling for shampoo commercials, gently smiles down at her baby. The chubby baby smiles back with just the cutest little hint of drool emerging from his gummy grin. Their eyes are locked in love and bliss. This, truly, is what motherhood is all about.

I've got news for you. One of the best kept secrets in maternity is that for 20 per cent of mothers (one in five) things are very different. She is deeply miserable, desperately tired, anxious and frightened, and the baby does nothing but scream abuse at her. Somehow her life seems to be coming apart at the seams.

Very often she tells nobody and nobody has a clue. Her parents and friends assume that as she has a healthy baby, she must be perfectly happy, and she is too ashamed to disillusion them. Her girlfriend rings her and

the new mother tells her how happy she is and how well everything is going. They share a joke and she hangs up. Looking in the mirror, she realises it's three o'clock in the afternoon, she hasn't had a shower yet and is still in her nightdress. She looks around her. The house is a mess with dust, dirty laundry and unwashed dishes. She feels and looks 20 years older than she did a few weeks ago. Her partner called an hour ago — he has to work late for the fourth time this week and he won't be home until eleven and don't worry about dinner. Then the baby starts to cry again.

Before the baby, everything had been fine. She had a great relationship with her man, they were in love. She had a job that gave her satisfaction and a role in the world, and was capable and confident. Finances were tight but they never let it get them down. Then came the baby and everything started to go wrong...

Postnatal depression is a catch-all phrase. Though it generally does not include the normal baby blues (which the majority of women get to some extent), it takes in the more severe depressive mood changes which last much longer, and which enter and interfere with every aspect of normal functioning. It does not include postnatal psychosis.

POSTNATAL PSYCHOSIS

This is a frightening and, thankfully, rare disease in which the mother's sanity becomes unstable and she loses touch with reality. It is separate from and unrelated to postnatal depression. Depression is a disorder of mood which may also affect thinking and bodily functions; psychosis is a disorder of the thinking process itself. In this psychosis there is usually a past or family history of a mental illness during which the patient had no insight into the fact that there was a problem. In the throes of the disorder she may well be very depressed, paranoid or anxious. Conversely she may be wildly happy, active and feel euphoric. But the hallmark is the interference with normal thinking patterns so that she has delusions, hallucinations and other thoughts out of touch with reality. These thoughts can make her do strange things and possibly be a danger to herself and her baby. She requires hospitalisation and medication but will usually do well, recovering gradually over the course of months.

It is important to understand that this disease is not a severe form of depression and has nothing to do with the baby blues. Indeed this disease can strike suddenly and unexpectedly and is completely unpredictable. It is also very rare. So remember, even intense depression does not lead to psychosis. They are two separate diseases.

POSTNATAL DEPRESSION

Within this hidden disease of motherhood, there is a spectrum of severity from the mild and transient 'fourth-day blues' to the severest form which can be crippling to a woman's whole life and wellbeing.

It reveals itself in a range of feelings, any combination of which may occur.

Deep depression and misery. This is just what the name of the condition implies.

Anxiety. A previously-confident young woman can become anxious about everything — traffic, strangers, illness in the baby or herself, even household implements may seem threatening. It may be so prominent that it emerges before (or overshadows) the depression, and so completely incapacitating that the woman remains cowering and housebound and jumps at the ringing phone. She may get panic attacks in public places, causing her to overbreathe. The hyperventilation then causes physical symptoms of its own. She may be unable to sleep or her sleep is beset with nightmares. She may be terrified of harming herself or her baby and convinced she is going quite crazy.

Anger. It is not unreasonable for a mother locked into this cycle of depression and anxiety to turn her anger onto the person who has caused it all — the baby. Not surprisingly, this brings out strong guilt feelings and worsens the situation. There is often a lot of anger directed at the partner, too. After all, his life is relatively unchanged: he still goes out to work, still has his friends and leisure activities. Of course, now there is another mouth to feed he has very good reasons to do lots of overtime ... quite apart from the fact that his partner is behaving strangely and aggressively towards him.

Last and not least, she is angry at herself, and this destroys her self-esteem.

Loss of self-esteem. Our confident young woman, who is able to hold down a demanding and responsible job has now been brought to her knees by a mere baby. What could be more destructive to her self-esteem? Some mothers don't even know they have postnatal depression. They just feel responsible for the whole mess because everything appears to be of their own making.

Chronic fatigue. Nobody knows true fatigue like the new mother. Indeed, the hormones released by pregnancy and breastfeeding seem to interfere with the normal sleep/dream/wake pattern of the normal person. When chronically fatigued, nobody can think straight, and lack of sleep usually plays a big part in the generation and maintenance of the depression. The fatigue also makes it very hard to get anything done, housework is abandoned, meals are forgotten and life just becomes too hard.

CAUSES AND REASONS

We can list the numerous factors which make the possibility of postnatal depression increase. But none of these external factors can be called the cause. Most mothers have a mixture of intrinsic and extrinsic factors causing their depressive state.

Lack of sleep usually plays a big part in the generation and maintenance of the depression.
▼▼▼

Intrinsic factors

First and foremost, whether or not you will get the severer kind of depression depends on whether or not you have an inherent tendency towards it. In other words, how bad is your luck?

Some women seem to have an almost purely intrinsic type of depression. Everything seems to be going well and there seems to be nothing in their circumstances that might provoke depression. Then a few days after the birth the depression sweeps over them, enveloping them like a dark blanket. From pregnancy to pregnancy they recognise the early signs — these appear not to change unless they take medication. It may even arrive during sleep and external factors seem to play only a small role in its genesis.

Extrinsic factors

Most depressed mothers have this intrinsic tendency but also need provoking factors from the environment to start the process.

- Was the pregnancy or labour worse than expected?
- Was the baby up to expectations? The wrong sex? A fractious screamer?
- Did the breastfeeding work?
- What's in the mother's past history? Depression? Is she an anxious type?
- Were there fertility or obstetric worries?
- How does she get on with her mother? Her partner?
- How good were her self-esteem and coping skills before the pregnancy?
- How secure are the family finances?

And on and on. None of these factors is particularly important in itself but they all play a part in bringing down a mother once the vicious depressive cycle starts to turn.

Without the intrinsic tendency, though, many such factors may come together in a woman and she will feel no more than the baby blues and manage to escape major depression.

WHAT TO DO

Admit the problem

Accept that you have a problem which cannot and should not be ignored and is a disease state that needs treatment. If you had pneumonia you would accept that you needed medical care, treatment, help and support with the baby. This disease is just the same. You owe it to your baby, your family and yourself to treat it seriously and allow your helpers to treat it properly.

Talk about it

It's very sad, but one of the symptoms of depression is an inability to get things done. This interferes with the most important part of the treatment, which is seeing someone about it. It is most important to sit and talk to someone who knows the issues involved. There is no doubt that the earlier you seek treatment, the sooner you can get back to being contented and feeling better about yourself. Happily, nowadays, postnatal depression is being seen for the common disorder that it is and more and more early childhood centre sisters, general practitioners, obstetricians and paediatricians quickly recognise the importance of the problem and know where to refer the sufferer. For milder cases, the family doctor and self-help groups are usually enough. However, for more severe cases, there is no doubt that a visit to a psychiatrist can make all the difference. Unfortunately, many women feel that this stigmatises them as crazy, but nowadays this belief has no foundation. Not seeing a psychiatrist because of this feeling could mean cutting off a vital channel of help.

Get counselling

Remember, this disorder might be telling you something. It is often bringing to a head issues in your life which need resolution and won't go away without attention. Now is the time to address the problems in your relationships with your mother, partner or baby. It is a time to look at what you expect from your family and your life. Try to make this time of unhappiness work for you to improve the quality of your life when you emerge on the other side.

Get some help with the baby. Perhaps your partner can take some time off work to give you a hand — it will also help him understand how tough it is looking after a baby. Perhaps you have an extended family you can call upon to lend a hand. If there is no-one, admission to a mothercraft hospital might ease the load for a while.

Join a self-help group

For this problem, sharing your experiences and difficulties with others in a similar situation can be very helpful and reassuring. There are postnatal depression groups in most population centres and your early childhood centre nurse or family doctor will know how you can contact them.

Take antidepressant medicines (if that is what your doctor recommends).

Remember that feelings of depression and anxiety are generated by our brains not only in response to external events but also due to internal chemical imbalance.

Do not overextend yourself, or have too high expectations of your ability to function.

▼▼▼

*The
awareness
that one is just
depressed —
not depressed
about
something —
can be a
comforting
aspect often
not realised.*

▼▼▼

Depression is as much a disease as pneumonia. In both, an abnormal process is triggered off in the body and various medications can help the body overcome its disease. Antidepressant drugs restabilise the correct chemical balance within the brain and this elevates the mood. If you are breastfeeding, it is unusual for these drugs to pass in any important quantity into your milk but check this with your doctor. The tricyclic anti-depressant drugs, monoamine oxidase inhibitors and anti-anxiety drugs in particular are not excreted in any appreciable quantity in breast milk.

Consider stress management

Postnatal depression is also a disease of stress. Hence stress management tools can be used to control it.

Firstly, use time management. When confronted with a major task, such as housework, break the task into small, bite-sized pieces and lay out a reasonable, realistic timetable to get the work done. Do not overextend yourself, or have too high expectations of your ability to function.

Secondly, learn to relax in a formalised way. Buy a relaxation tape, learn meditation or use breath control methods to try to get control of your anxiety.

Thirdly, take time out from the baby. Feed him, change him and put him in his cot and go for a walk in the garden or listen to some music. No baby has come to harm because his mother takes ten minutes time out for a quiet cup of coffee.

IN CONCLUSION

Here is a little gratuitious psychobabble that can be helpful because it happens to be true.

The brain's function is to think and generate feelings and it does so as a response to chemicals within itself. We are at the mercy of these substances in our day-to-day lives. Think about it. Under almost exactly similar circumstances, sometimes we feel happy, sometimes we feel sad, day by day. When we feel unhappy, we normally look for a reason in our lives to justify the feeling. That is, we attempt to find a 'hook' upon which to hang the emotion we feel. On another day, under exactly the same conditions, we may feel contented, and we then choose to ignore the same hook, which is still there.

Of course events can and do change our mood. The point is that we do not necessarily have to accept the emotion and all the thoughts that go with it as valid and important. We could instead just watch it as dispassionately as possible and accept it for what it is, a chemical imbalance, a ripple on the surface of our lives.

Easier said than done,

especially when the emotion is a very powerful and intense one, such as depression. Nevertheless, stepping back from our feelings for a moment and replacing the thought 'I feel just terrible about my life' with the more accurate 'I feel depressed and a little anxious' is a useful way to of identify the raw individual emotions and remove the justifying thoughts that surround and support them. This reduces their power over us. Also the awareness that one is just depressed — not depressed about something — can be a comforting aspect often not realised. Recognising that our anxiety is free-floating rather than attached to an object or condition in our life can be a step towards controlling the hold this emotion has over us.

What to do

Admit the problem

....

Talk about it

....

Get counselling

....

Join a self-help group

....

Take anti-depressant medicines
(if that is what your doctor recommends)

....

Consider stress management

....

CHAPTER 6

THE CIRCUMCISION DECISION

The procedure continues to have vocal advocates and critics both within medicine and without.

Most of us are aware that circumcision is an ancient Jewish ritual dating back to the time of Abraham, but few of us realise that the Jews were not the first to practise it. Carvings on the walls in the Temple of Karnak depict Egyptian priests over 6,000 years ago performing circumcision, making it probably the oldest surgical operation known. Many diverse cultures continue the practice today.

In modern times circumcision became extremely popular between the wars — especially in the USA and Australia and rather less in the UK. The influential American paediatrician, Benjamin Spock, though not wholly recommending it, thought that 'it made a boy feel regular' as virtually all boys in that era were circumcised.

But times are changing. Nowadays, in the city obstetric hospitals over 70 per cent of male babies are going home still complete with foreskin — often to the dismay of their grandparents.

With an ancient practice like circumcision it is not surprising that numerous myths have sprung up describing the results. Circumcision 'weakens the penis' and therefore limits intercourse (so said a 12th century rabbi); increases (others say decreases) sexual pleasure; decreases sexual desire; prolongs ability to have intercourse (in the act and in life); makes men better warriors and better husbands; reduces masturbation and cures bed-wetting. These claims are difficult to research, as you can imagine, but all are unreasonable and defy common sense.

Nowadays, we like to think we are more reasonable in our beliefs. However, the procedure continues to have vocal advocates and critics both within medicine and without.

Professors of urology argue with paediatricians, family doctors in the cities argue with those in the bush, surgeons argue with psychiatrists. Outside medicine the discussion gets even hotter among action groups such as the American NOCIRC (National Organisation of Circumcision Resource Centers) and INTACT (International Organisation against Circumcision Trauma) which have members who have undergone plastic surgery to reconstruct the foreskin and psychotherapy to relieve the psychological stress sustained by its removal.

The essence of the discussion remains simple. Does the latest information on the subject justify routine circumcision on babies? For other invasive baby routines, for instance immunisation or the administration of vitamin K, the benefits are so overwhelming and the risk so small that it's no contest. Circumcision, however, is entirely another matter. The question is, should we routinely subject a baby, or any minor who can't give his personal consent, to a procedure whose benefits are not proven or substantial, and whose risk is not negligible, to remove a piece of his body whose function is not clear?

THE FUNCTION OF THE FORESKIN

Logically, it seems likely that the foreskin has some function. Most of our other useless organs have been discarded by the process of evolution or remain only in a shrunken, vestigial form. Not so with the foreskin, which remains as large as life. Microscopic examination of the cells which are on the inside of the foreskin shows that it contains many sensory nerve endings relating to sexual excitation. In addition, the other nerves of the foreskin are numerous and similar to normal skin — hence they can discriminate fine touch, texture, warmth, and stretch. Not so the skin of the tip of the penis — this is relatively insensitive to warmth, touch and texture.

It would therefore seem reasonable, if the foreskin were being removed for social reasons, to obtain the permission of the owner. At the age of 20 he should be able to make an informed decision. Moreover it is totally wrong to suggest that circumcision hurts more at that age. In fact it is not a particularly painful operation — as long as one has a general anaesthetic and there is no postoperative arousal!

It is certainly an advantage for a newborn to keep his foreskin, as it affords protection for the penile tip or glans from the effects of nappy rash and it will preclude meatal ulceration, a small painful ulcer which develops at the opening of the urethra only in the circumcised.

Another common reason given for circumcision of the newborn is that the foreskin causes urinary obstruction. This is almost never the case and if it occurs at all it must be incredibly rare. Certainly, ballooning of the foreskin on passing urine is a normal finding and is certainly not an indication for its removal.

WHEN THE FORESKIN DRAWS BACK

A common reason given for circumcision in a baby is phimosis or narrowing of the foreskin. Many people — sadly including many medical and nursing professionals — are not aware that in the majority of baby boys the foreskin is not retractable. Only in 4 per cent of newborns can the foreskin

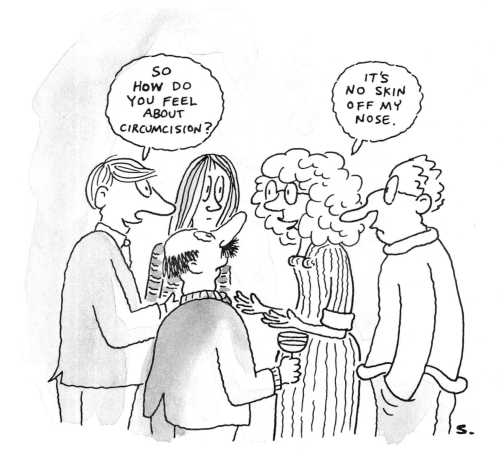

be fully retracted. As time passes the foreskin gradually separates from the underlying tissue, but still by 3 years of age there are 10 per cent of boys whose foreskin cannot be retracted. In these boys, as there is no space between the foreskin and the glans, no secretions collect and consequently there is no need for this area to be washed.

After the foreskin becomes retractable, such secretions do tend to accumulate and regular hygiene is necessary. Many misguided people forcibly retract the foreskin of the infant before it is ready and this causes tearing of the tissues and hence scarring and the subsequent possibility of narrowing (phimosis). This then makes retraction and normal hygiene extremely difficult. In fact, to correct this situation, circumcision may subsequently be required. Most people who recommend circumcision have gruesome tales of close friends or relations who had 'years of infection, pain and worry' from a foreskin that was too narrow until they were liberated by circumcision. One wonders how many of these poor men were suffering from a consequence of obsessive early retraction and penile cleansing when things would have been better left alone.

Some recent studies, however, have provided a bit more balance to the circumcision argument. Firstly, a study of the medical records of babies born in US Army hospitals has shown an increased incidence of urinary tract infection in those who were uncircumcised. The incidence of infection was still very small (about 1 in 600 babies) but this was ten times the rate for the circumcised. There remain some theoretical criticisms of the study, so the conclusion is not yet proven, but as other similar studies seem to have arrived at the same conclusion, it is likely to be true.

It is still open to debate that the possibility of urinary tract infection justifies the routine circumcision of every baby; for instance, the incidence of appendicitis is about the same (1 in 700 per year) but we do not recommend routine appendicectomy. Certainly this new information has not changed the stance of the American Pediatric Association, which is still firmly against routine circumcision.

The second study concerned sexually transmitted organisms. During sexual activity there is always the possibility of small breaks occurring in the foreskin when it is stretched around the glans. These breaks can allow easier access to some organisms (such as herpes, warts and HIV) that typically enter by way of such cuts in the skin. It has been claimed that having unprotected intercourse with an HIV-positive person is eight times more risky if one is uncircumcised than if one is

Many misguided people forcibly retract the foreskin of the infant before it is ready.

▼▼▼

*Parents often
believe that
circumcision
of the
newborn is
the 'normal
thing to do'.*

▼▼▼

circumcised. This sounds logical and reasonable. However, using a condom in this situation is a good deal more sensible than getting a circumcision.

It also seems to be true that cancer of the penis hardly occurs in the circumcised. But the incidence (less than 1 per 100,000, which is really rare) seems to be the same in the uncircumcised who wash themselves. Again, not a powerful argument unless your family are congenitally lazy in the bathroom!

THE PARENTS' DECISION

By far and away the most common indication for circumcision in the newborn period is parental preference. Parents often believe that it is the 'normal thing to do'. A father often wishes his son to be 'done' so that his penis and his son's penis look the same, lest any differences cause the boy upset and confusion. A child, however, will accept differences with far greater equanimity than would an adult, and the major difference between father and son, that of penile size, remains until the boy is well into puberty anyway. If the boy has brothers who are circumcised most parents seem to want a matching set, though again there is no evidence that differences cause any psychological harm.

THE SAFEST TIME FOR CIRCUMCISION

A very important question, one which is only infrequently asked by parents, is what is the safest time for a baby to have the operation of circumcision. The answer to this is the later the better. One thing is quite certain, the neonatal period (the first four weeks of life) is precisely the time when it is least safe. The newborn baby has immature immunity which makes him less than fully capable of fighting an infection should bacteria enter from his wound site. In addition, his clotting mechanisms are immature.

Most babies get jaundice in the first few days of life and one of the reasons for this is immaturity of the liver. One of the functions of the liver is to process the jaundice and eliminate it from the body. Significantly, clotting factors are also produced by the liver. It certainly seems illogical to trust the clotting mechanism of a baby who has demonstrably immature liver function. The only advantage of circumcision in the newborn period is that as the baby is so small, he can't fight back. It is felt therefore, quite unjustifiably, that no anaesthetic is necessary. Nevertheless, it is still much safer to have an anaesthetic and a circumcision in a paediatric hospital at a few months of age than it is to have an unanaesthetised neonatal circumcision.

CONSEQUENCES

It is general knowledge in the paediatric community that occasionally babies die as a direct result of circumcision, with at least 16 babies dying each year in the UK.

Other complications also occur. In a random study of a thousand families in England it was found that 22 per cent of the boys circumcised had developed some complication from the procedure, including haemorrhages severe enough to require transfusion.

It must be said, however, that despite the risks associated with the age group of the patient, the operation would be a good deal safer if it was taken more seriously. Too frequently it is delegated to the junior member of an obstetric team. The operative area has a very good blood supply and luckily heals very quickly and it is difficult for an infection to gain a foothold. Also the skin is very mobile and if too much is removed usually this makes very little functional difference, so most irregularities in technique are of no consequence. Nevertheless it is obvious that this part of the bodyis of tremendous psychological importance so if mistakes are made, the scars remain not just on the body but also in the mind.

It is much safer to have an anaesthetic and a circumcision in a paediatric hospital at a few months of age than a neonatal circumcision without anaesthetic.

▼▼▼

CHAPTER 7

SETTLING IN

Throughout the whole wonderful experience
of getting to know your baby
do not forget two very important people
— yourself and your partner.

Most first-time mothers can't wait to get home after having their babies. Significantly, most second-time mothers have to be prised out of their hospital bed and sent home, kicking and screaming! There is a lesson here for first-timers. Remember, not only does the housework await you, but when your friends visit they now expect to have a cup of tea and wake the baby for a cuddle. They usually stay too long, too.

There are a few things to consider before going home. Your anxiety level about your baby is likely to increase. Also, you will tend to rush around a lot more so it is likely that you will be more tired, so your breast milk supply will diminish slightly over the first day or two. The combination of these factors is likely to make your baby behave differently for a few days and this can make both your anxiety and your fatigue worse.

My advice therefore is to expect a change in your baby's behaviour and accept it. Remember that his behaviour changed from day to day in the hospital and will continue to do so at home until a pattern is established. In addition, ignore the housework, or get dad to do it, and rest as much as possible.

SIBLINGS

Imagine how it must be. You are two years old and the supreme ruler of your family. One day your parents bring home a baby, a young pretender to your throne, and mummy, your personal slave, starts giving this intruder a lot of attention. And to add insult to injury, he regularly sucks on her breasts, which up to now have been your private property.

Your plan of action:

- Become a baby again — demand a dummy and require a daytime nappy.
- Do everything in your power to divert mummy, especially during feeds.
- Be as naughty as possible — after all, any attention is better than none.

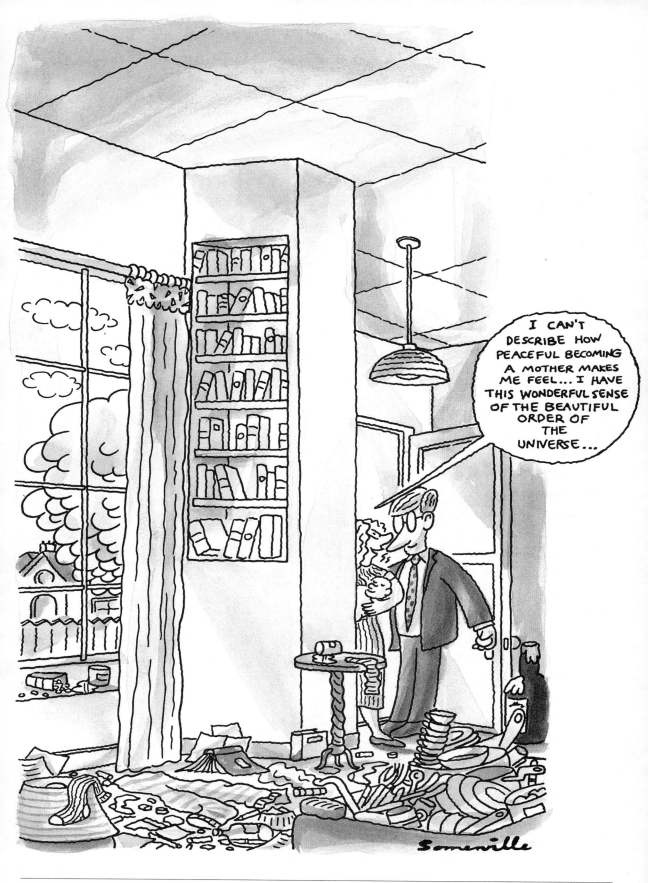

Bringing home a new baby heralds a major lifestyle change for a hitherto only child and this has to be sympathetically appreciated and planned for by mum and dad.

In the hospital, make sure that all the baby's tasks have been done before the older sibling comes at visiting time. This will allow you to spend all your time and attention on the older child. If the baby cries or plays up, try to ignore the baby or leave it to dad.

When the time comes for you to leave the hospital, big sister or brother should come to help you take the baby home, but should hold your hand while dad carries the baby. The worst thing you can do is send the older child away to grandmother when you bring the baby home, in the mistaken belief that it will smooth your return. You will be sending the child a clear message about whom you now prefer.

Use your common sense and make looking after the baby a joint project. Give the older child a baby doll of his or her own to look after, and get the child to help with the baby — even if each task takes twice as long. Shower the older child with affection. Try to make him or her feel responsible for their little baby. If both are crying at the same time, try to comfort the older sibling first.

Siblings under 20 months do not seem to mind a newcomer as much as those over 20 months; and the nearer the child is to three, the easier this will be. But two-year-olds are trouble.

FRIENDS

For the first few days after you go home, your real friends will stay away — or if they do show up, they bring dinner! As for the others, do not wake the baby for them. Be polite but firm and give them some housework to do. It is to be hoped that they will remember an urgent appointment.

SLEEP

Next to feeding, sleeping is the subject that most concerns new parents (their own as well as their baby's!).

The normal baby's requirement of sleep varies enormously. Studies show that the range lies between 10 and 23 hours per 24 (with a 'typical' baby sleeping about 16 hours per 24) in the first week after birth. This period shortens only by an hour or so during the rest of the first year but the pattern changes. Young babies sleep almost as much during the day as the night, but as they get nearer to six months the night-time sleep gets longer and the daytime naps become fewer. It is futile to worry if your baby seems to sleep for only short periods of time. The babies who sleep for 23 hours a day and awaken only for feeds are usually other people's babies. Some babies may spend most of the daylight hours watching their mother, blinking at the light and generally enjoying all the activity around them. Of course there is the other crowd who don't like to nap, but when they are awake, they whinge. Other babies sleep during the day and howl all night.

Generally speaking, tired babies sleep. If it's not enough for you, try the manoeuvres in the chapter 'Colic and the Crying Baby'. Be reassured that no baby has ever become sick from lack of sleep — only his poor parents have.

The question of where the baby should sleep is worth a little attention. Though the family bed has its fans, I'm not one of them. It's inconvenient, disruptive and has no proven psychological advantages. Indeed, a study showed that children in our culture (important emphasis) had a much higher incidence (up to 50 per cent!) of sleep problems at five years old when the family slept in one bed.

How about the baby's cot next to your bed? Certainly for some mothers it is a good way to go if he's a frequent feeder during the night, just hook him in to bed and get on with it. For a few mothers, for a few weeks only...

But mostly I would suggest that it is a good idea to have the baby sleeping in his own room right from the early days. Babies are often noisy sleepers, grunting and groaning, pushing and straining. This is invariable in premature babies by the time they go home and it is for this reason most neonatal intensive care units suggest that the mother spends the night with the baby before she takes him home. She normally returns to the unit in the morning wide-eyed with sleeplessness and surprise at the symphony of noise that her baby has made all night.

Full-term babies can also match the ex-prems for noise and as long as the parents don't think he is straining because he is constipated they will soon see that it is a normal phenomenon.

Many babies also have an interesting breathing rhythm where they pant for a while, then stop breathing for up to nine seconds before starting to pant again. This pattern is normal in the first three months of life, but it is a rare parent who can listen to it and get any sleep. By the end of the nine seconds they are usually wide awake and halfway to the cot.

So move the cot to the baby's room — you spent all that time decorating it, now use it!

It is a good idea to have the baby sleeping in his own room right from the early days.

▼▼▼

NAPPY RASH

The sensitive skin of a newborn baby can be prone to a number of problems, mostly minor ones.

Remember, dermatologists' and paediatricians' babies get nappy rashes too. It does not reflect upon the quality of your care of the baby.

Nappy rashes can be divided into three general types:

CONTACT RASH

This rash occurs in those areas in contact with the nappy, leaving the creases of the thighs unaffected. It is mainly caused by irritation of the skin, from moisture in the nappy and also by substances in the urine, like urea, forming ammonia after being broken down by germs from the baby's stool.

Treatment. Wash the nappies in commercial preparations such as Napisan and rinse them carefully, or try disposables for a week or so. Stop using soap on the skin and use a nonsoap cleanser with pine tar instead. Use a cream containing zinc and castor oil at first, but if there is no improvement, see your doctor. He or she may prescribe 1 per cent hydrocortisone cream to use at each nappy change. Once the rash has improved, use a silicone-based barrier cream to protect the skin.

RASH IN MOIST AREAS

This rash tends to be worse in the creases of the skin, though it may be uniform throughout the nappy area.

Treatment. Use the same management approach as for the contact rash, but in this case the rash may be caused by thrush. See your doctor, who may prescribe some 1 per cent hydrocortisone cream and Vioform or some other antifungal antiseptic such as Daktarin cream.

If either this rash or the contact rash refuses to go away, stop using lanolin (in moist towelettes or baby lotions, for instance) altogether.

EXCORIATED BUTTOCKS

This rash occurs around the anus and is usually from the stool. The stool of breastfed babies is very acid, and, especially if the stool is frothy or fluid, can burn the buttocks.

Treatment. Frequent nappy changing, exposure to the air and 1 per cent hydro-cortisone cream should improve matters. A silicone-based barrier cream will protect the skin.

ECZEMA

This characteristic rash occurs in mild form in many babies, usually in the first four months of life. The skin of the cheeks becomes rough and scaly and scaliness of the skin under the hair and eyebrows, called cradle cap, develops. In severe form, the baby can have scale, cracking, weeping and redness caused by infection to the skin of most of his upper body, especially behind the ears, back of the neck, face and chest. The condition is caused by overactivity of the sweat glands and the treatment is directed to diminishing their activity. Babies usually grow out of this tendency in the first six months.

Occasionally, in families that are atopic (that is, families that have an allergic tendency), this kind of rash tends to last for longer — even blending into adult-type eczema as the child grows.

Treatment. Stop using soap for bathing. Instead, use a nonsoap cleanser containing pine tar. If the rash is severe, limit bathing to a couple of times a week. Avoid the use of fancy baby lotions and creams. Moisturise the skin with sorbolene, with or without glycerin and use 1 per cent hydrocortisone in sorbolene cream from your doctor in all but the mildest cases. This steroid cream is very mild and perfectly safe for babies and may be used liberally. It is the mainstay of the treatment. Avoid the use of brushed synthetic fibres or wool next to the skin. If the rash is more than mild, it is best to have it treated by your doctor.

CRADLE CAP

Cradle cap responds well to petroleum jelly (Vaseline), which softens scales and allows their removal. It is worthwhile trying a tiny amount of antidandruff shampoo now and again, as this is also likely to help.

- Cradle cap is (seborrboeic) eczema of the scalp (or eyebrows).
- The mildest cases will resolve with sorbolene.
- If it is more severe, have it treated by your doctor — who will probably limit bathing.

UMBILICAL HERNIA

Some babies develop a swelling under the umbilicus that gets larger when they yell or tense up their tummy. If you squeeze it, it may gurgle and the contents disappear back into the abdomen. This is the one hernia in the body you can completely ignore. It never causes problems, doesn't ever burst, never strangulates and doesn't require

You can completely ignore an umbilical hernia. It never causes problems, doesn't ever burst, never strangulates and doesn't require surgery.

▼▼▼

When you go out in the summer, the baby should always have sunscreen on exposed skin and wear a hat or bonnet with a brim.

▼▼▼

surgery. It is just the small gap in the muscle layer of the abdominal wall through which the umbilical vessels to the placenta passed, and is composed of a very strong membrane. It will disappear gradually, and in the vast majority of babies is completely gone before the child reaches the age of five, and usually long before that.

UMBILICAL GRANULOMA

Sometimes after the cord falls off you might notice a wet, pinkish knob of tissue on the leftover stump. No matter how hard you clean it, it keeps weeping fluid and won't heal over. This can last for weeks and sometimes the lump even

gets bigger over time. It is called a granuloma and is due to the healing (granulation) tissue getting too enthusiastic and not allowing the normal skin to cover it. If you take your baby to your health nurse or doctor they will put on a little copper sulphate and it will rapidly disappear.

SUN KICKS

Sunlight should really come with a warning: 'This radiation is harmful to your health and, in sufficient dosage, may even be lethal.'

Sun kicks are quite helpful to those who live in the northern hemisphere, where the radiation is lower, or who have a diet short of vitamin D. It is not relevant somewhere like Australia, where

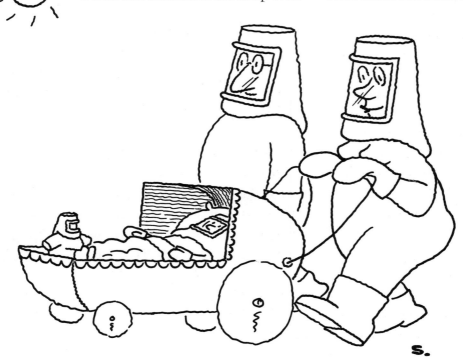

babies should be exposed to the naked rays of the sun as little as possible. When you go out in summer, the baby should always have sunscreen on exposed skin (the rumours about the 15+ lotions being harmful for babies are completely untrue) and wear a hat or bonnet with a brim. To see small babies sunbathing naked on beaches is a sad sight — quite apart from the long-term aspects of skin cancer, babies can burn badly in minutes.

The days of worshipping the sun are numbered. It will soon be fashionable to have porcelain skin (and no wrinkles until you're 60!).

ORAL THRUSH

Babies have relatively immature immune mechanisms and many of them are not able to withstand infection with a common environmental fungus called *Candida albicans*, which usually occurs in the mouth. The infection, better known as thrush, looks like white milk curds stuck to the inside of the cheeks. Unlike milk, though, they cannot be scraped off. They can also occur on the baby's gums and palate. Thrush can cause soreness but most babies are pretty tolerant of it and it should not cause a feeding problem.

The fungus can be removed effectively by Nystatin or other antifungal medicines (such as Daktarin gel) put in the baby's mouth after he has had a feed. It is also worthwhile putting some antifungal cream (such as Mycostatin) on your nipple if you are breastfeeding to stop cross-infection. If bottle-feeding, be very careful with sterilisation of the bottle and equipment. The thrush is never resistant to these antifungal agents; however, it is sometimes difficult to eradicate due to constant reinfection from the feeding equipment. So change the sterilisation fluid you use for dummies, bottles and teats even more often than usual until the infection starts to come under control.

REFLUX

'My baby vomits all the time and brings back everything I put into him.'

'Is he putting on weight normally?'

'Yes, but ...'

The mother of a baby who has (gastro-oesophageal) reflux can be recognised by her harassed expression, the nappy permanently on her shoulder and the smell of sour milk that accompanies her wherever she goes.

Frequent vomiting can be a demoralising nuisance. All that beautifully-produced milk dumped

Frequent vomiting can be a demoralising nuisance. Be reassured, the majority of babies will grow out of their reflux problem, usually in the first four months.

▼▼▼

I have never met a normal breastfed baby who was constipated, that is, passing hard stools.

▼▼▼

on the shoulder of your dress or saved for daddy's trousers when he gets home! The vomiting may be effortless or projectile and the baby is often hungry afterwards.

All newborn babies reflux to some degree. There is a valve that lies between the gullet and the stomach which works very poorly in newborns, so the milk may go up and down the gullet like a yo-yo following a feed. In some babies, it comes out of the mouth, in other babies it does not. If there is a problem with reflux, it starts when:

- the amount of vomiting becomes more than a nuisance;
- the baby does not put on enough weight;
- people start blaming the baby's crying on the vomiting, saying the baby has 'heartburn' (see the chapter 'Colic and the Crying Baby').

Be reassured, the majority of babies will grow out of their reflux problem, usually in the first four months. The question is — can you wait that long?

Initial treatment should be to adjust the baby's resting position. The best posture to empty the stomach and keep the feed as far away from the gullet as possible is with the baby right side down and head up at about 30 degrees from the horizontal. For really bad cases, it may be worth propping up the

Breastfed babies have an immunity to bacterial gastroenteritis

▼▼▼

head of the cot on blocks. Some doctors recommend the use of an antacid to decrease the irritation on the lower end of the gullet after each feed. If the reflux is bad in a bottle-fed baby, it is worthwhile thickening up the feeds with carobel or some other thickener. Later on, the introduction of solids can do the same thing. Your doctor can also prescribe some drugs, such as cisapride (Prepulsid) or bethanecol (Urocarb), which help close the valve between the gullet and the stomach, although these probably should not be first-line treatment.

Only in worse cases is an operation to make the valve more efficient necessary. This is extremely rare. Most babies (and their mothers) struggle through and the problem disappears.

BOWEL ACTIONS

BREASTFED BABY

For a breastfed baby it is normal, once meconium has been passed and the milk is in, for the baby to have 20 stools a day or one every two weeks. Anything between these two extremes is normal. The stool can be yellow, green, brown or any combination of these. It can be frankly fluid, seedy or pasty. For breastfed babies, it is never hard. I have never met a normal breastfed baby who was constipated, that is, passing hard stools. If you are worried that your baby has not passed a stool for several days, when he eventually does pass it, you can be reassured by its consistency. If it is anything other than rabbit pellets it is normal.

Breastfed babies who produce stools less frequently can seem uncomfortable on the day, or perhaps the day before they produce them. You will soon get to know your baby's particular patterns and accept this as quite normal. Breastfed babies never need any help to go more frequently.

The only stool that should cause you concern is when it is so watery it resembles urine. Under these circumstances it is wise to seek medical advice as the baby may have gastroenteritis. Breastfed babies have immunity to bacterial gastroenteritis, but viral disease can still occur (see below). The baby producing the loose frequent stools is often the baby who is spilling a little sugar of milk (lactose) in the stool. This is a normal finding and does not represent lactose intolerance.

BOTTLE-FED BABY

Bottle-fed babies tend to have rather firmer stools and to pass them between four times a day and once every two days. The colour tends more to the rustic browns and greens rather than the Van Gogh yellow. It is certainly possible for them to become constipated, but again, the diagnosis rests on the fact of hard stools rather than infrequency. If the stool is firm or hard, adding a little maltogen or brown sugar (one to two teaspoons to a bottle) or offering a small amount of prune juice will normally be sufficient to soften it. Sometimes well-diluted orange juice and extra water will be helpful. Don't be tempted to use suppositories for your baby unless you check with your doctor — it is almost never necessary.

DIARRHOEA

Loose watery stools in the bottle-fed or breastfed baby should be treated with respect as they might indicate the presence of gastro-enteritis. Even the fully breastfed can get this, specifically from a virus called rotovirus.

Unlike the normal loose stool of many breastfed babies, this stool is 'urine-like' and resembles water. If you're unsure, check with your doctor, as the main danger of diarrhoea in the baby is dehydration, which can occur rapidly due to their small reserves of fluid. But, if your baby is still wetting three nappies a day there is no immediate danger. Nevertheless, go and see your doctor anyway as this problem does need medical attention. Take a

Bottle-fed babies tend to have rather firmer stools and to pass them between four times a day and once every two days.

▼▼▼

sample of the stool with you. To collect one, line a nappy with a plastic bag so the fluid is also caught. If you have to wait very long for the stool, it's probably all right anyway!

Breastfed babies can usually continue feeding normally but bottle-fed might benefit from a change to a lactose-free formula.

OUT AND ABOUT

DRIVING

It is incredible the number of unrestrained children one can see in the back or, worse, the front seats of cars. These presumably loving parents are obviously unaware that with the slightest deceleration of the car their child becomes a missile so heavy that the strongest man could not hold on to him. Anyone who has worked in a children's intensive care unit for a short time will tell you of the agony of parents who are completely unharmed after a minor collision and whose child has gone through the windscreen and now lies broken or dying in hospital. No journey is so short that a child should be unrestrained. Remember, most road accidents occur within a short distance of home.

It is now mandatory by law that your baby must always travel in a restraint device in a car. The best one is a rear-facing safety capsule. Get it fitted as soon as, or before,

No journey is so short that a child should be unrestrained.

▼▼▼

you go into labour so that it is all ready to take your baby home from hospital. Quite apart from the safety aspect of the first drive home, it gets you into the habit of never having children or babies in the car unless they are fully restrained.

As your child grows, if he strongly resents being strapped in, then it is a very good time to teach him some discipline and for him to realise that some rules are unchanging and not open to negotiation.

Like child abuse, there is never any excuse.

FLYING

Airliners are pressurised to an atmospheric pressure equal to that at 5000 feet, so it is perfectly safe to take even your newborn baby to see his relatives overseas. Beware only if he was born prematurely and had severe lung disease.

It is, in fact, a good deal easier to travel with a newborn baby than it is with a toddler. Babies do not have the constant need to move around and can usually be comforted with the breast or a feed. They also do not kick the chair in front, spill every drink handed to them, need to go to the toilet only when the food trolleys are blocking all the aisles or become fascinated with the hair of the man in the seat in front.

Pressure problems in the middle

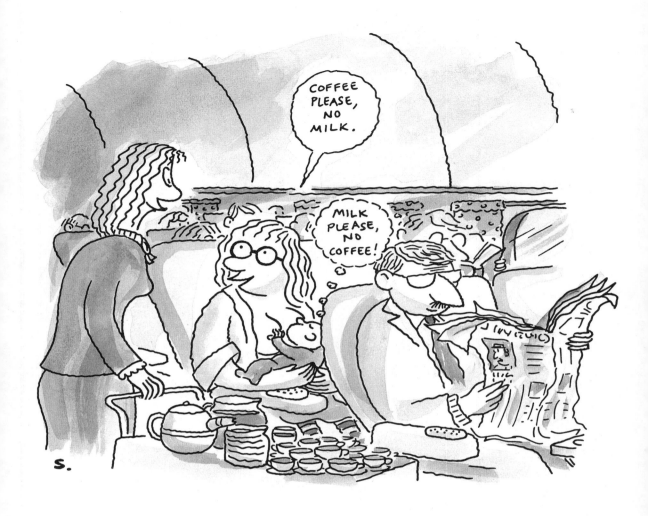

ear on descending are probably less common in babies than they are in adults, as the Eustachian (connecting) tube between the pharynx and the middle ear is much shorter. Nevertheless, when the plane descends, it is worthwhile getting the baby to suck, as this will equalise pressures around the eardrum. Unfortunately, pilots do not always tell you when they start their descent, which is often an hour before arrival, so be ready.

Strictly speaking, it does not really matter if the baby becomes upset because of the pressure in his ears because he will yell and that is precisely the best treatment to equalise the pressure. His noise should not worry your fellow passengers as their ears will also be affected by the descent!

It is a good deal easier to travel with a newborn baby than it is with a toddler.

▼▼▼

WHEN TO CALL THE DOCTOR

Babies have countless ways of worrying their parents and it is important at these times to remember that there is a great range of normal behaviour. All new parents are naturally anxious about their baby's health, and it is easy to overreact. On most occasions, no intervention is necessary. However, if your baby exhibits any of the following signs or symptoms, get your doctor to check things out.

Use a baby paracetamol elixir to control a high temperature. Temperatures over 38°C should be treated with respect, and the baby taken to a doctor for diagnosis.

▼▼▼

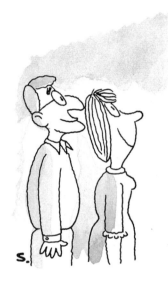

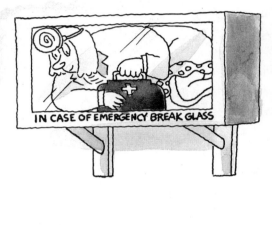

IN CASE OF EMERGENCY BREAK GLASS

- Baby's respiratory rate is 60 or more per minute maintained over five minutes or more;
- Baby's temperature is greater than 39°C (102.2°F) or below 36°C (96.8°F);
- Fits or convulsions;
- Fewer than two wet nappies per day;
- Increasing jaundice beyond one week of age;
- Blood in stool or urine beyond one week of age;

- Baby is pale and listless;
- Baby refuses all feeds;
- Combination of vomiting and watery diarrhoea;
- Repeated projectile vomiting;
- Symmetrical red inflammation around the base of the stump of the umbilical cord;
- Baby has difficulty breathing;
- Barking seal-like cough;
- Baby does not move limbs symmetrically;
- Baby doesn't look right.

FEVERS, COUGHS AND COLDS

Newborn babies who are breastfed rarely get infections of the upper respiratory tract (coughs and colds). There are antiviral substances within the breast milk that have a protective effect. Indeed, in the case of middle ear infection, the effect seems to last even after the baby has been weaned and even if the breastfeeding only lasted a few weeks. That is not to say that the baby will not develop snuffles (see section on 'Snuffles').

Having said that, it is still possible for your baby to catch a cold, especially if the baby's older brother or sister is going to playgroup or preschool and bringing home all the viruses that are going around. If your baby has snuffles and a temperature then it is probably due to a viral infection. The normal underarm temperature for your baby is 36.5°C (97.7°F). Any temperature over 37°C (98.6°F) is probably significant. The management of a cold, 'flu or a mild cough is purely to treat the symptoms. There are no antibiotics or drugs that can kill viruses. We must wait until the baby's immune mechanism fixes the problem by itself.

But, to control a high temperature, a baby paracetamol elixir is very useful and may be given in the correct dosage (15 mg/kg body weight) for the baby's age, every four hours. This dosage must not be exceeded. If the baby has a blocked nose bad enough to interfere with feeding, a drop of nasal antihistamine decongestant can clear it for long enough to get a feed down. Nasal decongestants should not be used regularly, however, except under medical advice. Anyway, it is a good idea to have your doctor check to make sure there is no middle ear or chest infection.

Temperatures over 38°C (100.4°F) should be treated with respect and the baby taken to the doctor for diagnosis. If there is also a diagnosed viral illness, the temperature will continue to stay high, and the baby should be treated with paracetamol elixir regularly. If this is not enough, sponging with lukewarm water helps to bring the temperature down. Do not use cold water, as it is less effective in extracting warmth from the baby's body. To take the baby's temperature, use a mercury or digital thermometer under his armpit or the stick-on ones for his forehead.

Respiratory viral infections normally right themselves in a few days but if your baby develops a wheeze, a seal-like bark or a 'smoker's cough' see your doctor straight away.

Newborn babies who are breastfed rarely get coughs and colds.

▼▼▼

COT DEATH

Nothing strikes fear into the hearts of parents quite like cot death — sudden infant death syndrome (SIDS). Luckily, however, it is really quite rare. About 2 in 1000 babies are lost in this unexpected and insidious way. By definition, the babies die quietly, without a struggle, during sleep and on careful examination of the circumstances and the baby, no cause can be found.

Statistics tell us that it more commonly occurs in boys than girls, during cold months rather than warm months of the year, and in bottle-fed rather than breastfed infants. It occurs maximally between the ages of two and four months and the majority occur before six months. It is rare after one year.

Maternal factors can play a part — there is a slightly increased incidence if the mother smoked cigarettes and a larger increase if she was addicted to narcotics or barbiturates in the pregnancy. There may be an increased chance of SIDS in the siblings of those who have died in this way.

You can paper the walls with theories as to the cause, but basically it probably comes down to a failure of the breathing drive. Feeding into this final common

SIDS — WHAT YOU <u>CAN</u> DO

- Think about it as little as possible.
- Buy an intercom (a simple wire one is not expensive, a radio transmitter type will cost more).
- Get your baby used to sleeping on his side or his back and position his lower shoulder forward so if he rolls, he rolls onto his back, not his front. Don't worry about the baby sleeping on his back, it's perfectly safe. Babies are not like coma patients who might inhale stomach contents if they vomit. Even flat on their backs babies are perfectly capable of looking after their airway if they vomit. I'm afraid it was neonatologists that started the vogue of sleeping babies on their fronts in the first place, as it has some advantages to the premature, but there are no such advantages in the full term.
- Avoid nonporous, too soft mattresses. Babies don't need or like pillows.
- Make up their bedding so their feet can touch the bottom of their cot. This gives them some control so they don't disappear down under the covers, possibly causing overheating or suffocation.
- Avoid overwrapping your baby with blankets or warming his room too much, especially if he has a cold or other infection. An ideal room temperature is about 18°C (64°F).

pathway are many factors, some genetic, some not, and nobody has yet come near to satisfactorily unravelling the web of these combining factors to explain all cases. Nevertheless, these factors are worth noting, even at our present level of knowledge.

- The front-down or prone posture of an infant in the cot seems without doubt to be less safe than that on the side or the back.
- Breastfeeding, to a degree, seems to be protective.
- Smoking during pregnancy is an added risk factor.
- Overheating of the baby (caused by a fever, too warm an environment or overwrapping) may contribute.

Though clearly these are not anything like causes or explanations they are definitely worth noting and acting on, to minimise the risks as much as possible.

MONITORING

No-one has shown satisfactorily that the electronic monitoring of babies makes any difference. Some babies fire off the alarm because they stop breathing, but no-one knows whether they would have gone on to die if left alone, or whether this 'apnoea' (Latin for 'no breathing') attack is even the same condition. Also, babies still die of cot death while being monitored — by the time the monitor alarm goes off, many of them cannot not be revived.

We all share the same fear — paediatrician and printer, bus driver and journalist. Every parent whose baby first sleeps through the night will remember the hollow feeling in their stomach as they walk towards the baby's room to check that their baby is still breathing. As already mentioned, it is not worthwhile electronically monitoring babies who have no special risks. There are usually too many terrifying false alarms and the monitor is no guarantee of preventing SIDS. For very anxious parents a monitor may decrease the anxiety and for those it is an option to discuss with the paediatrician. I have seen some parents who would otherwise have watched the baby in shifts and never slept together again until the baby was two, but such anxiety is rare.

It is likely that in the future we will discover that there is an inborn or intrauterine factor which increases the propensity for some infants to stop breathing in this way and the external factors just trigger the event. Research is now underway in many centres to find such a inborn error and hence a screening test. Until that day comes, just keep on remembering that the danger of SIDS is less than that of being run over when you cross the road.

Remember, the danger of SIDS is less than that of being run over when you cross the road.

MOTHER NOT MARTYR

Throughout the whole wonderful experience of getting to know your baby in the first few weeks, it is critically important that you do not forget two very important people — yourself and your partner. It takes some effort to juggle everyone's needs and take care of yourself at the same time in this situation. Eat normally and regularly. If you are breastfeeding, your weight should diminish anyway as you transfer your fat deposits to the baby and it is important to have a good nourishing diet to provide for you both.

If you are obsessive about

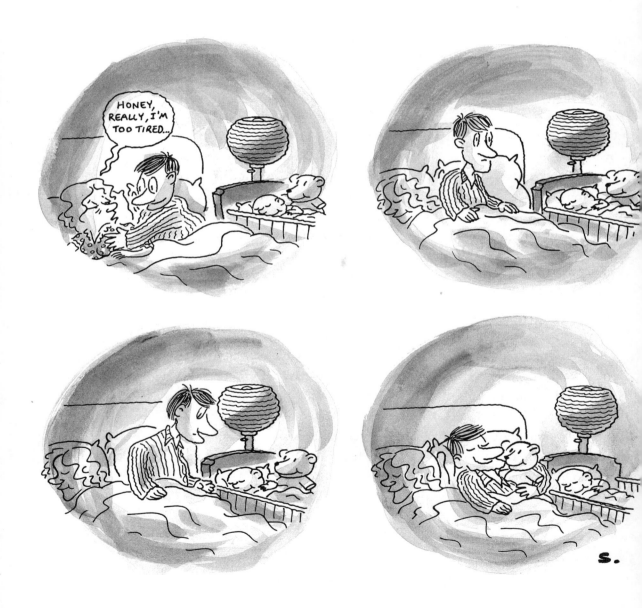

housework, try to get some help. This is no time to clean, wash and scrub. If you can't get help, let the house go just a little and enjoy the little spare time you have.

As fathers have not gone through delivery, they may not fully understand that it takes some weeks for you to recover your strength, quite apart from the nocturnal demands made on you by a little baby. Sex may be the last thing on your mind in these first weeks, but do not forget that it may be uppermost in your partner's. The most vital sexual activity for you both at this time is to talk about it and not just avoid the subject. Then when your libido starts to return you don't find a cranky, jealous mate who feels he's been jilted in favour of a baby.

Babies have a few critical needs and the most important is a happy mother and father in a stable and loving relationship. This aspect of baby care needs as much attention as nappies.

In fact, don't be surprised if recovery takes longer than you expect. A follow-up study of over 400 mothers found that sexual problems such as decreased libido, discomfort with intercourse and difficulty reaching orgasm reached their peak at three months after the delivery with four out of ten women affected. And half of these continued to have these problems for over a year.

The study also showed that though many of the physical problems were resolved in the first month, breast problems, haemorrhoids, dizziness, fatigue, hair loss and constipation sometimes persisted for between three and nine months after delivery.

It takes some effort to juggle everyone's needs and take care of yourself at the same time.

TIMETABLE OF DEVELOPMENT

BIRTH

At birth your baby lies on his front
with both his knees tucked under
his abdomen with his head to the
side. He tries but cannot lift his
head off the mattress. If you turn
him over and pull him up by his
hands (it's quite safe), his head lags
backwards. He has active
'primitive' reflexes. If you tickle the
palm of his hand, it will clench in
the grasp reflex. If his head is
allowed to flop backwards, he will
demonstrate a well-developed
startle (Moro) reflex in which he
throws his arms out. If he is held to
stand, he will make clumsy walking
movements with his feet, although
this is sometimes hard to elicit. He
can't yet turn to sound but will gaze
fixedly towards the light.

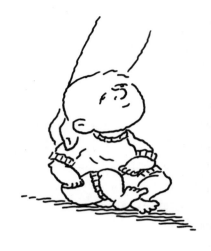

FOUR WEEKS

At four weeks he intermittently
attempts to raise his head from the
mattress and, on being pulled to sit,
has a little head control. His grasp
reflex is still present but his other
primitive reflexes are starting to
disappear. He will now follow your
face through a narrow arc, and in
the next week or so, he will start to
smile back at you if you smile at
him first.

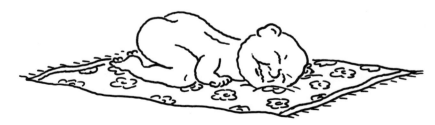

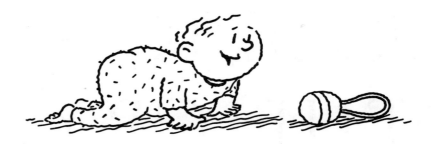

EIGHT WEEKS

At eight weeks he can lift his head off the mattress when on his front, and his head control is much improved. He has now lost his grasp and walking reflexes and only part of his startle reflex remains. He can clasp his hands in the midline and can put them in his mouth. His eyes fix and focus and he can follow you with his eyes through a wider arc. He is starting to chuckle and coo.

TWELVE WEEKS

At twelve weeks he can look up when lying prone and even push himself up with his hands. When he is pulled to sit, his head is very stable, with only an occasional wobble. He starts to notice his hands and will hold onto a rattle which is placed in his hands. He turns his head towards sound and recognises his mother. He has even started to babble conversationally.

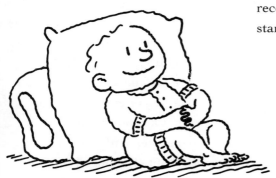

CHAPTER 8

COLIC AND THE CRYING BABY

There is no doubt that colic exists.
In most cases the basic cause of the whole problem
is tension, anxiety or stress in the baby.

Whenever a baby cries for no apparent reason and won't stop, it is likely to be labelled 'colic' or 'wind'. Even more so if his legs are drawn up to his tummy as he yells, if he passes a lot of wind, or, if picked up, he can be burped.

If the bouts of crying start occurring frequently, parents usually notice that a pattern emerges and start searching frantically for a cause. Then comes the avalanche of advice. It is incredible to hear the advice given to these poor unfortunate parents; everything from 'tummy massages', 'a drop of brandy' to the saddest suggestion of all, 'put him on the bottle'.

All useless, all untrue, but frantic, tired parents are an easy target for these 'helpful' people.

There is no doubt that colic exists, because at its most severe, descriptions of events from different parents are remarkably similar. It tends to recur at certain times of the day, most commonly in the evening — hence 'six o'clock colic'. During the attacks the baby appears uncomfortable and squirms, drawing his knees up and crying or even screaming with apparent pain. Occasionally he will waken out of a deep sleep with a 'jump' and this will precede a bout of crying. The smallest thing can trigger off the attacks — passing wind, wetting his nappy or just 'being bored'. Sometimes they occur around feed times with the baby pulling off the breast and screaming.

The attacks may be relieved by picking him up, cuddling and feeding, or vigorous sucking on a dummy. Occasionally the baby will calm down when he is driven around in a car but often nothing helps at all.

Not surprisingly, the situation can create enormous domestic tension. There is something about the incessant crying of a baby that drives even the most even-tempered people up the wall. Soon both parents are at the end of their tether, sleepless, frustrated, angry and guilty. Guilty about the anger they feel at this ungrateful little being, for whom so much is being done for so little reward.

At the outset it is important to realise that most of the old beliefs about colic are just myths, and acting by them often makes matters worse.

Firstly, babies who cry will swallow air. The wind does not cause the crying — the crying causes the wind.

Secondly, colicky babies and their parents are perfectly normal people, without special allergies or psychological problems — except those caused by a baby screaming at them for a few weeks!

Thirdly, in nearly all cases there is nothing whatever the matter with the baby's tummy. Any baby who gives a vigorous cry is liable to draw his knees up — this gives a bit more power to the yell, it is not that he's got a pain. When one thinks about it, it is quite illogical that a breastfed baby, fed with the most

physiologically pure food available, should develop a tummy ache from it. Nature is usually a bit more efficient than that! Also, parents often notice that the crying is worse at a particular time of the day — often the evening. As babies are fed on a 24-hour clock it is unlikely to be the fault of the feed or his tummy.

There is a newer scapegoat. Heartburn from gastro-oesophageal reflux (see 'reflux' page 89) is often now given the blame, and treatment with antacids or other more high-tech medicines such as cisapride is recommended. However, radiologically-proven refluxing babies mostly do not suffer colic; indeed, most babies can be shown to reflux in the neonatal period.

Screaming babies are also liable to reflux as they tense their tummy muscles and increase the pressure in their abdomen.

If the baby has a bit of lactose intolerance (see page 63) and has loose stools and a gurgly tummy, then usually this is blamed for the 'pain'. However, there is an equal number of comfortable babies with similar stools, and research studies are far from convincing.

Indeed, whatever the colicky baby does that is 'not average' will be blamed for the noise: if he feeds a lot, or a little, if he has loose or firm stools, or if he screams when he wets his nappy.

So the breastfed baby does not

There is something about the incessant crying of a baby that drives even the most even-tempered people up the wall.

▼▼▼

Whatever the colicky baby does that is 'not average' will be blamed for the noise.

▼▼▼

All over the world, in different climates and cultures, babies are typically unsettled between four in the afternoon and nine in the evening.

▼▼▼

need the bottle and the bottle-fed baby does not need his formula changed. Neither does he have distension or spasm in his gut. All these particular myths have been perpetuated through history because of the baby's appearance and behaviour, and you can't blame anyone for being fooled.

It is worth knowing that all over the world, in different climates and cultures, babies are typically unsettled between four in the afternoon and nine in the evening. So what is the connection between babies in Australia, Guatemala, India and the USA?

It is fairly certain now that in most cases the basic cause of the whole problem is tension, anxiety or stress in the baby.

WHY SHOULD A BABY BE TENSE?

When the baby is in the womb he gently floats around in a sea of warm, soothing water in perfect peace. Following delivery, things are very different. His life is now more noisy and active. He has hunger, thirst, discomfort and fatigue. His posture is no longer contained, secure and snug. He is no longer a physical part of his mother. Some babies may find all of this very hard to tolerate, and they react accordingly.

On top of the abrupt life changes, there is an additional compelling factor that causes babies to be subject to stress. Research with premature babies has shown that they (and to a lesser extent term babies) are very susceptible to overstimulation. Things such as noise, activity, disruption or stress in the home atmosphere may arouse and stimulate a baby. However the most powerful stimulus is human contact, and, especially, eye contact.

Think about how we usually approach a baby. Most people gaze deep into his eyes and make noises to attract his attention and get him to gaze back. Unfortunately, a lot of such intense eye contact can be very stressful for a young baby. It really excites him. It would be all right if he could just switch off the input, as older people do, when he has had enough. Alas, babies just can't do this. They are excited and 'stressed' and they cry. This is one clear explanation for this problem occurring more in the evening.

When a baby cries it is normal and appropriate for his parents to become anxious and concerned about him. We know from research that a baby's cry is imprinted into his mother's mind within a few hours of birth. His cry then acts as an 'arousal mechanism' over which she has little control. It is not only normal for a mother to become agitated and to wake out of the deepest sleep when her baby cries,

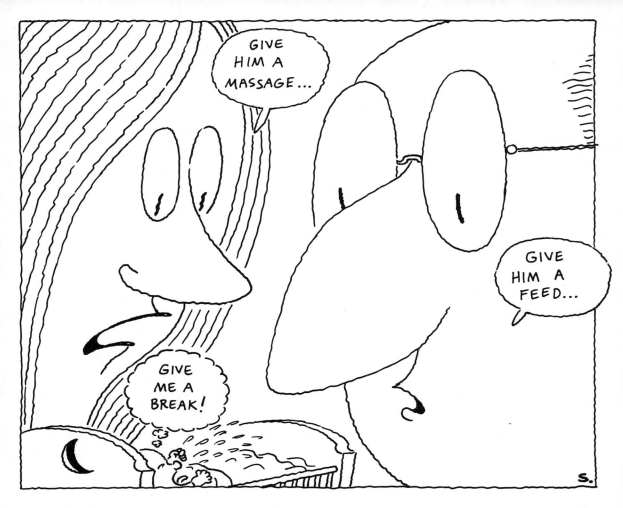

it is a fundamental survival reflex for the baby. This maternal instinct sends the mother into a frenzy of activity, finding out what is wrong and meeting the baby's needs to stop him crying. But as babies are very sensitive to stress from their surroundings, this very activity can make them more anxious and make them cry even more. This makes the mother more anxious, more active and makes her cry more. Round and round the vicious circle goes, driving both into intense anguish and misery.

Even more directly, the parents' response is often to go to the baby, pick him up, look him in the eyes and ask him what the problem is. This is like putting the rock music back on and the baby just keeps dancing! What he is really saying is 'Please leave me alone!' and that is precisely what they are not doing.

Clearly, some babies are better at coping with such stimulation than others. The variable is the baby's personality. Some babies can cope, and others can't, at least for a few months, until they learn to switch off.

Most babies will grow out of this problem by about four months of age. So hang in there!

Research with premature babies has shown that they are very susceptible to overstimulation.

▼▼▼

WHAT DO WE DO ABOUT IT?

In the early stages it is often enough for you and your partner to realise what is going on to control the problem. If you realise that, if anything, there is too much parenting rather than too little in your family and the baby's cries don't represent intense agony, pain or a rejection of your love, then you are more able to think straight about the problem.

First, listen to your baby's different cries. I'm sure there are several. A hungry one (loud and insistent), a tired one (mumble, mumble, bleat), need a cuddle (waa, waa, waa), and so on right through to the mind-wrenching scream of the overstressed, anxious or insecure baby. Try to sort them out and 'tune in' to what's behind them. Stop a while and think before reacting. Get to know your baby's other signals. Hiccupping is commonly a sign of a full stomach but sometimes is a sign of agitation and stress. Yawning, straining and pushing with the limbs are signs that the baby may be overloaded with stimuli and would prefer a period of peace and quiet.

If there's any possibility that the cry may be a hungry one, feed him. If you're wrong, he may not be interested or may vomit: it doesn't matter either way. You'll know next time and it's important to eliminate this cause of crying before you move onto other things. Overfeeding is not a problem in the short term, so don't worry about it.

Once that possibility is out of the way, you can turn to more subtle things. Try to make your infant feel as snug and secure as possible. Swaddling is a good technique. It works even better if the wrapping persuades the baby to lie like a fetus, with the back rounded and head forward slightly, shoulders hunched, arms and legs flexed towards the body. This gives the baby a sense of security. The swaddling should be firm enough so the hands, shoulders and legs are all contained. Lying the baby on his side whilst swaddling will also help to encourage sleep.

Hold him until he relaxes. Often these stressed babies resist the swaddling and fight to get their arms and legs free so they can flail them around. This is very upsetting for them and should be resisted. Gentle but firm persuasion should keep the limbs contained in the blanket. To calm him use dim lights and a gentle voice. Avoid too much eye contact and don't overload him with your voice, rocking and looking at him all at once.

Once he settles, place him on his side or back in his cot and, at an early opportunity, vacate the area. If he starts crying again, don't go in straightaway but see if he calms

Some babies are better at coping with stimulation than others.

▼▼▼

down by himself. If he does not, repeat the swaddling and calming, soften his environment as much as possible by relaxed, slow movements and again leave as soon as he settles.

It is critical to understand that it is all right to leave the baby once he has settled a little. If he has been fed, changed and cuddled and still he continues to cry, then it is best for him that you don't get 'sucked in' any further.

Remember that the function of crying in the human is that of a de-stresser. You feel bad, you cry, you feel better. So it is with your baby; it may be just what he needs to calm down.

From here on you should do whatever calms you the most. If that is to carry him around — that's all right. But equally, if it is to leave him in his cot to cry and get yourself a stiff drink, then that's all right too.

There comes a time when you know that your presence is not helping. Indeed, you may find that when you pick him up he will stiffen and his cries will increase. He is saying 'Please leave me alone, I've had enough for one day!' Don't hover outside the door wringing your hands, as he can sense you out there. Try to get out of earshot for a while, before going back to check on him.

How long you leave him depends on two things — him and you! If he starts really screaming again, go in and calm him before settling him again on his own. If you find it difficult not to go in when your baby cries, leave him for ten minutes or so before going in to check on him. When you go in, don't turn on the light, and avoid eye contact with him.

There are other techniques worth a try:

- Relaxation baths will often calm down an excited baby. The water is ideally about 20 cm (8 in) deep and the usual warm temperature. Instead of bathing the baby on his back and supporting the back of his head, which allows his arms to fling out as he startles, float him on his front with a hand under his chin to keep his head out of the water. The water must be deep enough so he does not touch the bottom, but floats gently on the surface. Many babies promptly go to sleep when immersed in this way.
- Carrying babies around in a pouch often provides a comforting environment for the brittle-tempered baby, allowing him to be held against his mother's chest while leaving her arms free. Babies usually calm rapidly when carried this way.
- If the baby finds comfort in sucking, let him. Whatever your prejudices about dummies, this is one situation when they should be buried.

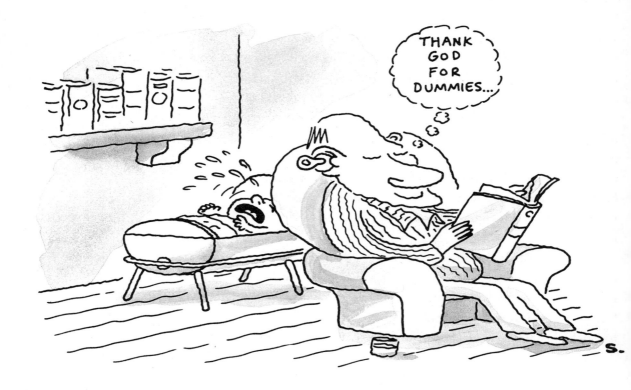

An important fact to remember is that no young baby has ever damaged himself, either physically or emotionally, from crying.

▼▼▼

- For dog-tired parents, help from a third party can give them the sleep they so badly need to get their confidence back and allow a more balanced view of the situation. So ask grandmother over for the weekend — she may enjoy being needed, despite the noise.
- Sometimes a small dose of sedative for the baby will help to calm him. (When anticolic medicines work it is because they are sedatives.)
- Moving mother and baby to a residential mothercraft home, if one is available, almost always solves the problem.

The lesson of self-calming (clinical psychologists call the process 'returning to base') is an important one for a baby to learn in the first few months of life. When he is calm he can then get on with the next task, that of learning to concentrate.

The only other important fact to remember is that no young baby has ever damaged himself, either physically or emotionally, from crying. Whatever else they are, babies are superbly designed crying machines who can, and occasionally do, cry for hours nonstop without harming anyone but their parents!

WHY YOUR BABY CRIES AND WHAT YOU CAN DO ABOUT IT

WHAT IS MAKING OUR BABY CRY?

The truth:

- wind does not cause the crying — crying causes babies to swallow air;
- colicky babies (and their parents) do NOT have special allergies or psychological problems;
- there is almost never anything wrong with the baby's tummy;
- heartburn (from gastrointestinal reflux) is not usually the cause of the crying; and
- lactose intolerance, feeding a lot or feeding a little are not the cause either!

> **ALL OVER THE WORLD, IN DIFFERENT CULTURES AND CLIMATES, BABIES ARE TYPICALLY UNSETTLED BETWEN FOUR IN THE AFTERNOON AND NINE IN THE EVENING.**
>
> **THE BASIC CAUSE OF THE PROBLEM SEEMS TO BE TENSION, ANXIETY OR STRESS IN THE BABY.**

Noise, activity, disruption or stress in the home environment may stimulate a baby. The most powerful stimulus, though, is human contact, especially eye contact. Picking up the baby and looking deep into his eyes when he cries is probably going to make matters worse, not better!

WHAT WORKS?

1. Listen to your baby's different cries and learn their meanings — hungry, tired, need a cuddle, through to overstressed, anxious or insecure.
2. Try feeding the baby — it's an easy problem to solve, or you can eliminate it from your list of possibilities.
3. Make your baby feel snug and secure — swaddle him, keeping his hands, shoulders and legs contained.
4. Hold him close until he relaxes — use dim lights, a gentle voice, and not too much eye contact.
5. When he's relaxed, put him in his cot and leave. If he starts crying again, go back to swaddling and calming.
6. From here on, do whatever calms YOU the most!

Other techniques to try:

- relaxation baths
- carrying the baby around in a pouch
- letting the baby suck
- help from a third party — giving yourselves a break
- a small dose of sedative
- a stay at a residential mothercraft home

> **REMEMBER, NO BABY HAS EVER DAMAGED HIMSELF, PHYSICALLY OR EMOTIONALLY, BY CRYING. AND MOST BABIES WILL GROW OUT OF THIS PROBLEM BY ABOUT FOUR MONTHS OF AGE. SO HANG IN THERE!**

CHAPTER 9

IMMUNISATION

*Immunisation is one of the
greatest boons from medical science
in the history of humanity.*

It's very hard to believe that there are people around who believe the world is flat. You can show them maps, even pictures from space, but they still go on believing their nonsense. It is a similar story with immunisation. There is a body of people who never waste an opportunity to push their belief that immunisation is useless or even harmful. The media are often to blame for publicising tragedies coincident with immunisation and inappropriately laying blame. This only reinforces the biases of the ignorant.

The anti-immunisation lobby bases much of its argument on the fact that in the West, infectious diseases were generally on the wane before the introduction of immunisation. This was usually because of improvements in hygiene, sanitation and nutrition. But this doesn't detract from the enormous impact immunisation programmes had, independent of these environmental improvements.

Make no mistake. There is an overwhelming and vast body of evidence that shows that immunisation is one of the greatest boons from medical science in the history of humanity.

Let's outline all the individual immunisations your baby needs and have a look at the evidence that makes doctors, nurses, public health officials (and most parents) very enthusiastic about them being available for every baby.

MATERNAL ANTIBODIES

Firstly, at birth, babies have the same antibodies as their mother, transported to them across the placenta. If she is immune to chickenpox or measles or tetanus — from having had either the disease or the appropriate immunisation, then so is her baby. This is called passive immunisation and it lasts from three to six months for most diseases. After this the level of antibodies falls to such a level that they can no longer protect the baby. Hence the need for the active immunisation that is the subject of this chapter.

THE TRIPLE VACCINE AND THE SABIN VACCINE

At eight weeks it is recommended your baby has the first of a series of three injections to prevent him getting diphtheria, tetanus and pertussis (whooping cough). He will also be given an oral vaccine to prevent him getting poliomyelitis. These vaccines will be given at two months, four months, six months and eighteen months, though the timing varies somewhat from country to country.

DIPHTHERIA

In the past this was a real killer. For instance, in the 1880s it carried off about 14 per cent of toddlers in South Australia. In 1890 passive immunisation with an injection of the antibody to the germ's toxin reduced the incidence by 50 per cent but even so, just before World War II, 300 people in Australia were still dying from the disease each year. Then, around that time, active immunisation with the diphtheria toxoid was introduced and the disease all but disappeared.

The germ of diphtheria lives in the soil and dust and can infect the skin directly. However, the more common form is a severe throat infection and is spread by contact with the droplets in a cough or a sneeze. Death can result from suffocation or more commonly by heart failure caused by the toxin produced by the germ.

Immunisation aims to give protection against the toxin. This is achieved by giving inactivated toxin (toxoid), which causes production of antibodies.

TETANUS

Tetanus is another extremely nasty disease lurking out there. The spores of the disease are common in our environment, ready to pounce on us if we drop our guard. Tetanus is a frequently fatal disease caused by the poison produced by the tetanus bacillus. This germ grows if it gains access to deep tissues, usually through a penetrating (but often very small) wound in our body. The toxin causes muscle spasms and organ failure.

It is still a common cause of death of babies in the Third World, where the organism gets access through the umbilical cord (occasionally from tribal customs such as putting animal dung on the umbilical stump). Many babies in developing countries are now being saved by active immunisation of the mother, whose antibody is then transferred to the baby through the placenta during the last few weeks of pregnancy.

Tetanus immunisation works very well in the individual and lasts

At birth, babies have the same antibodies as their mother. This passive immunisation lasts from three to six months for most diseases.

▼▼▼

At eight weeks your baby should have the first series of three injections to prevent him getting diphtheria, tetanus and pertussis (whooping cough).

▼▼▼

a long time. However, unlike the situation with contagious diseases, the risk of disease in unimmunised individuals is unaltered by the high level of immunisation in the community. It is purely our own and our children's responsibility. Also, we all need to have our antibody level boosted by a booster immunisation every ten years. Again, the immunisation is with a toxoid, similar in mechanism to diphtheria.

PERTUSSIS

Pertussis (or whooping cough) is a respiratory tract infection usually occurring in children and characterised by paroxysms of fitful coughing and the production of sticky, gluey mucus. The cough so empties the lungs of air that following the coughing spasm there is a 'whoop' as the air is sucked back into the lungs. It is a serious and prolonged illness in children (in China it is called the 'hundred-day cough') but it actually kills babies. This is because they often have the disease without the characteristic cough but have attacks where they just stop breathing.

The vaccine consists of killed bacteria and is effective in 80 to 90 per cent of cases. This is enough to prevent the spread of infection. In public health jargon it improves 'herd immunity', that is, it reduces the reservoir of people who are harbouring the germ at any time and therefore reduces the opportunity of spreading it to others who are vulnerable, such as babies.

The vaccine has, unfortunately, been a public relations disaster. It is this component of the triple vaccine which causes most of the mild and major side effects. And it is this vaccine which led to the erroneous belief that vaccination can cause permanent brain or neurological damage. Of all the vaccination tragedies that hit the papers the pertussis vaccine is usually carrying the blame.

In the United Kingdom before the 1950s there were about 100,000 notified cases of pertussis each year, with numerous deaths. By 1973, following the enthusiastic introduction of a vaccination program, 80 per cent had been vaccinated and the number of cases had dropped to a little over 2000 cases a year.

Then two factors emerged. Firstly, people thought whooping cough had been defeated and stopped fearing the disease, forgetting that it was a killer. Secondly, publicity about the side effects of the immunisation started to become more prevalent.

Consequently, immunisation rates fell, and by 1975 only 30 per cent of the population were immune. The country paid the price. In 1978 and 1982 there were

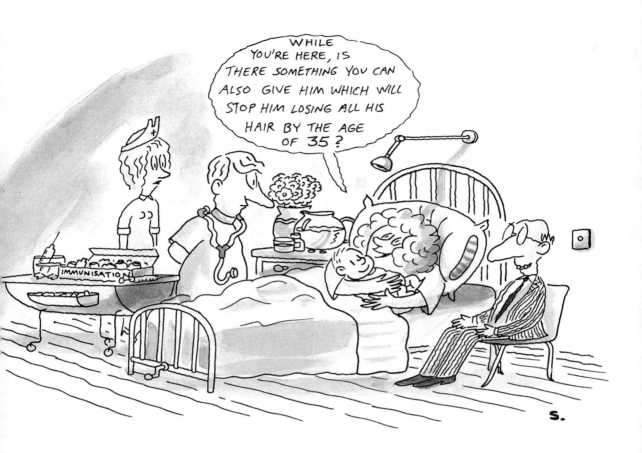

epidemics, each of which had over 65,000 cases and about 30 deaths.

There were similar experiences in Sweden and Japan.

These experiences of pertussis immunisation in England and elsewhere demonstrate graphically the most powerful arguments against those who would not immunise. Nobody could argue that environmental conditions, general nutrition or hygiene (the usual reasons given by anti-immunisation groups to explain falling disease rates) were relevant to the impact of the immunisation program.

The epidemics were solely a consequence of the increase in the number of children who were at risk of getting the infection (that is, a fall in herd immunity). This was a direct result of complacency, scaremongering and the fear of what are, in fact, minimal side effects.

On receiving this immunisation about half of the babies will manifest some side effects. Usually this is only a small local reaction, a red weal or swelling at the site of injection. Babies may also get a mild fever or be a bit whingey for a few hours. This complication rate can be halved by the administration of

In Britain, when rates of immunisation dropped to 30 per cent, there were two whooping cough epidemics.

▼▼▼

paracetamol, 15 mg/kg given to the baby at the time of the injection and every four hours (if the baby is awake) for three or four doses.

However, a small percentage of children will have side effects a bit more worrying. 1.5 per cent of children may get a fever over 40°C (104°F), 1.1 per cent of children may cry for more than three hours and 0.6 per cent will have a hypotonic/hyporesponsive attack. In this they become floppy and apparently unconscious. Even more rarely they can get shock reactions and even a brain swelling. Luckily these are extremely rare.

Of importance is the fact that none of these reactions, frightening though the rare ones are, cause permanent damage to the baby. As so many babies are being immunised, it is likely that there are some who have gone on to develop brain injury, fits or even cot death, from whatever cause. It has merely been assumed that the two were related: that is, that the pertussis vaccine caused the problem. This has been shown by the most exhaustive and extensive studies to be completely untrue.

The National Collaborative Perinatal Project (USA) investigated the incidence of fits following the immunisation. It found that by chance alone two out of every 10,000 children would have a fit within two days of any given time. They then studied the

two days following the immunisation and found that only 1.5 children per 10,000 actually had a seizure. Therefore, if it happened it was coincidence.

An even more detailed study, the National Childhood Encephalopathy Study (UK), looked at the incidence of permanent brain disorders following immunisation. It came to a provisional (and much publicised) conclusion that the chance was 'less than 1 in 310,000', but since the original publication the data have been re-examined in even greater detail and the present estimation is that the risk is 'virtually zero'.

To sum up, nobody has found any relationship between immunis-ation and permanent neurological disorders. Naturally, however, if a baby is diagnosed as having a neurological problem following an immunisation it is easy for a journalist to write an emotive story which blames the immunisation and plucks at the heartstrings. Looked at scientifically and properly, the relationship just isn't there.

The same can be said for the relationship between immunisation and cot death. By its very nature, cot death leaves the parents and friends looking for a cause, and if the baby had been immunised in the previous few days, it is a logical, though incorrect, relationship to make. But there is no relationship, no connection between the two.

Let us hope that the unbalanced media publicity and the scaremongering of the pressure groups are not too influential. Because if these things adversely affect immunisation rates, there will be an increase in the number of deaths from the immunising diseases. Remember, even with intensive care and modern technology, the death rate from pertussis can still be as high as 1 in 300 of babies who catch it.

POLIOMYELITIS

This was one of the few diseases that became more common once living conditions improved in the developed world. This is because if poliomyelitis is contracted as a very young child, as occurs in under-developed countries, it usually causes no problems. However, when acquired for the first time later in childhood or in early adult life, it can lead to paralysis.

Consequently, during the 1940s and 1950s there were epidemics in the West, and in Australia there was widespread panic and social disruption as the disease took hold. The disease led to an average of 100 deaths per year.

Poliomyelitis is a gut infection caused by viruses which invade the nervous system. It is passed from person to person by bad hygiene or poor sewage. The first vaccine developed was called the Salk vaccine, and was made from killed polio viruses which, when injected, caused the formation of antibodies in the blood. This vaccine cut the disease rate by 99 per cent after the first year of introduction.

Later, with mass screening programs using the oral (Sabin) vaccine, the disease has virtually been eliminated from the developed world. The Sabin vaccine contains strains of living polio viruses that have been 'attenuated' or 'inactivated'. Given orally, this virus establishes itself in the bowel, causes the formation of antibodies in the lining of the bowel and in the blood of the recipient, thus preventing later infection by the wild infective type of virus. It works very well, many babies being immune following their first dose. A full course of three doses will produce long-lasting immunity in more than 95 per cent of people.

A word of caution. Oral polio vaccine is extremely safe; but, if the recipient's immunity is not working efficiently, for any reason, it should not be given. For instance, it should not be given to those receiving immunosuppressive drugs (including radiation), or cortico-steroids (except as cream on the skin) or to patients suffering from lymphoma, leukaemia or tumours of the immune system. The Salk vaccine should be used for these patients instead. The Salk vaccine should also be used for babies who

The oral (Sabin) vaccine works very well, producing long-lasting immunity in more than 95 per cent of people.
▼▼▼

TO VACCINATE, OR NOT TO VACCINATE?

IT IS **OK** TO VACCINATE IF THERE IS:

- A local reaction from the previous dose that is less than 5 cm across.
- A fever after the last dose of less than 40.5°C (104.9°F).
- Recent exposure to, or convalescence from, an infectious disease.
- Mild infective illness.
- Current antibiotic therapy.
- Pregnancy of the child's mother or others in the household.
- A family history of convulsions, or sudden infant death syndrome. Also, a family history of significant adverse events following immunisation.
- Static neurological disease (such as cerebral palsy) or even progressive neurological disease. Naturally, a doctor's opinion should be sought. The reason such diseases have been contraindications in the past is the fear of the normal progression of the disease being blamed on the immunisation.
- Prematurity. Premature babies should be vaccinated at their chronological age, that is, counting from the time they were born not corrected for their prematurity. That is because premature babies' immunity starts to mature as soon as they are born.

DON'T VACCINATE IF FOLLOWING PREVIOUS IMMUNISATION THE BABY HAD:

- Convulsions.
- Encephalopathy (swelling of the brain), even though this condition invariably gets better.
- Persistent screaming for three hours.
- Collapse or shock-like state.
- Fever greater than 40.5°C.

are returning to households where there are people with the above conditions, as the live attenuated viruses could be passed on to them.

Breastfeeding does no harm to the vaccine and is not a contraindication to its administration.

CONTRAINDICATIONS TO VACCINATION

A recent Sydney study showed that 16 per cent of children seen in a children's hospital casualty department were over a month late for their vaccinations. This happens because many people want babies and children to be in perfect physical health before they are immunised, so even a cough, sniffle or minor temperature causes the immunisation to be delayed. This is not in the best interests of the baby. In fact there are very few true contraindications to vaccination and unless the baby has got a real illness or is obviously actively fighting an infection (as manifested by a high fever) he should have his immunisations on time.

NEWER VACCINES FOR BABIES

HEPATITIS B

This virus causes liver disease and occurs commonly worldwide. It causes an acute liver inflammation in older children and adults, about 5 per cent of whom become long-term carriers of the virus.

Infected infants rarely get the acute hepatitis, but most of them become carriers. Carriers are a danger to others, as a source of the virus, and to themselves, as they have an increased risk of chronic liver disease or liver cancer.

The virus is transmitted by exposure to blood, and other body secretions (especially sexual) from an infected person.

The most common transmission of this virus globally is from those mothers who are carriers of the disease to their babies, around the time of delivery. It is important that these babies be immunised at birth to prevent them becoming carriers and so perpetuating the disease.

For the older child, although some authorities recommend this vaccination at the moment, nobody has been able to prove scientifically that there is a danger of babies and children catching hepatitis B 'horizontally', that is, from other adults or children with whom they play or live, in the normal course of events.

The hepatitis B virus can cause chronic liver disease.

▼▼▼

The disease becomes a danger later, when sexual activity begins, or if intravenous drug-taking starts. So definitely get all adolescents immunised before the age of sex, drugs and rock'n'roll — like 12 years old. However, if you want to protect your child (younger than 12) against the possibility of a needle-stick injury from a drug addict's syringe on the beach, then get him immunised earlier. The vaccine is completely safe and the program is for three injections, starting anytime from birth onwards, the second one a month later and the third six months after the first.

HAEMOPHILUS INFLUENZAE TYPE B (HIB)

Tears of joy stung the paediatric community's eyes on the release of a vaccine that really works against HIB disease. This nasty little bug is the commonest life-threatening bacterial infection in Australian children between the ages of one month and five years. It causes invasive infection in 1 in about 300 children. Of these children, about 20 die and an equal number are left with a severe handicap.

When children are very young (under the age of two) this germ tends to cause meningitis which can kill or cause brain damage. There is a particularly high incidence in the Aboriginal community in babies

under six months of age.

As children get older (between two and five years old) this germ then gives them a disease called epiglottitis (incidentally, they are not immune from this even if they have had the HIB meningitis). In this disease there is extreme swelling of the soft tissues at the top of the throat which causes respiratory obstruction, asphyxia and death unless the child receives intensive care quickly. Children can also get infections of the skin, joints and bones.

Now that we have effective vaccines, this disease will, we hope, become one of only historical interest in the countries that have immunisation programs. There are several so-called conjugate vaccines against HIB available and they are all effective; however, babies require at least three doses in the first 12 months (plus a booster at 18 months) to become immune. This is another of those infections where herd immunity is important, as there is a reservoir of this germ in our community, mostly in the under-fives themselves. In the USA this disease is called the 'day care' disease, as the more children a small child meets the more likely he is to meet someone with the germ. However, some countries such as Finland have completely eliminated the disease, even though not everybody was immunised, by building up enough herd immunity

The most common life-threatening bacterial infection in Australian children between the ages of one month and five years is HIB.

▼▼▼

and gradually eliminating the reservoirs.

These vaccines also cause very little in the way of side effects, either local or general. However, if your baby gets a local reaction to the first dose he is less likely to get one with his second or third. Don't hesitate to get this immunisation!

MEASLES, MUMPS AND RUBELLA

At 12 to 15 months of age your baby will be due for his measles, mumps and rubella immunisation. In some countries they give it earlier — at nine months — and then give a booster later.

MEASLES

Measles is a highly infectious disease. During the infectious stage, which lasts three weeks, vast numbers of viral particles are excreted in the respiratory secretions and these have a high likelihood of infecting any unimmunised person. Consequently, even with high immunisation rates in the population, epidemics can still occur. But, for those who are immunised, the vaccine is very effective. For instance in the USA the number of measles cases was reduced from 3.3 million to 3500 per year by an immunisation program in the early 1980s. Don't be misled by your own experience: measles is not a trivial disease. In the Third World it causes over 1.5 million deaths each year and even in developed countries neurological and respiratory complications still cause handicap and death.

If your baby is exposed to measles before being immunised, make sure he gets the immunisation then and there. In concert with the antibody given him from the placenta at birth it will provide adequate protection.

MUMPS

Mumps is less contagious than measles and it generally infects older children and adults. Nevertheless, it is the commonest viral infection of the nervous system with 15 per cent of mumps sufferers having signs of meningitis. Luckily, this is usually self-limiting, and sufferers completely recover. It also commonly causes inflammation of the testicles and infertility in postpubertal males. Immunisation works very well. In the USA between 1967 and 1983 there was a 98 per cent decrease in notifications following a vaccination program.

If your baby is exposed to measles before being immunised, make sure he gets the immunisation then and there.

▼▼▼

The vaccine for measles, mumps and rubella should be given at 12 months of age and again in the early teenage years.

▼▼▼

RUBELLA

Rubella (German measles) is a relatively minor infectious disease which causes illness with fever and a mild rash in most people. On the fetus, however, its effect is terrible: rubella damages the fetus and causes congenital malformations if the mother catches it during the first three months of her pregnancy.

The previous practice of vaccinating only young teenage girls still left a lot of virus among the young males, and this would infect any women whose immunity was not complete.

Immunisation programs are extremely effective but we need to achieve as near to 100 per cent compliance as possible, to remove the reservoir of virus in the population, and so totally eliminate this damaging fetal disease.

WHEN TO ADMINISTER THE VACCINE

The vaccine for measles, mumps and rubella is a mixture of live attenuated (inactivated) viruses. The vaccine should be administered at 12 months of age and again in the early teenage years. There are, however, some contraindications (see box below).

HOMEOPATHIC IMMUNISATION

Last but not least, there is absolutely no scientific evidence that so-called homeopathic immunisation bestows anything except a false sense of security.

CONTRAINDICATIONS TO THE MEASLES, MUMPS AND RUBELLA VACCINE

- Severe infective illness.

- Hypersensitivity to neomycin or kanamycin. If your child is allergic to eggs it doesn't necessarily mean he cannot receive the vaccine. However, it should be done under the supervision of an immunologist.

- Previous anaphylactic (severe allergic) reaction.

- Impaired immunity.

- Pregnancy.

- Injection of immunoglobulin in the previous three months.

Immunisation schedule

2 months   First dose of DTP (triple antigen), Sabin (polio) vaccine and HIB vaccine.

4 months   Second dose of DTP (triple antigen), Sabin (polio) and HIB vaccine.

6 months   Third dose of DTP (triple antigen), Sabin (polio) and HIB vaccine.

12 months   Measles, mumps and rubella vaccine (MMR).

18 months   Fourth dose of DTP (triple antigen), and HIB vaccine.

5 years   Pre-school booster — diphtheria tetanus (DCDT) and Sabin (polio) vaccine.

Immunisation records
- Record all your baby's immunisation in the Personal Health Record, sometimes known as the 'blue book'.
- Acurate immunisation records will make it easy for your child to get an immunisation certificate at school entry.

CHAPTER 10

LOSING A LITTLE, LOSING IT ALL

*Following loss, the grieving and
the healing process
are the one and the same.*

To a greater or lesser extent, being delivered of a baby with a congenital malformation or, even worse, suffering the loss of a baby, sets in train the grieving process. Its function is to help us adjust and recover and go back to living our lives in fullness and contentment.

The first response to this kind of tragedy is often total disbelief. Our mind plays tricks on us, telling us that it is not true and that we will soon wake up and all will be well.

Alas, soon this numbness wears off, to be replaced by anger and sadness. We feel cheated that this could happen to our baby. We examine the pregnancy in minute detail to try to find a reason, and even though there often is none, the feeling of responsibility and guilt remains.

CONGENITAL MALFORMATIONS

About 4 in 100 babies are born with a congenital malformation, of which about half are serious and may threaten the life of the baby. It is a profoundly disappointing event and one that all prospective parents secretly fear. If the baby is seriously ill they also have to contend with the possibility that the baby may not survive. It is most important that the parents seek and get the maximum factual advice regarding their baby's problem as soon as possible. The nights will be long enough without needless fears caused by not knowing what is going on, or not knowing what his prospects are, or what surgery is necessary and when it should be done. There are a number of special advice and support groups for many of the more common malformations such as cleft palates, Down's Syndrome, or spina bifida; these groups can provide a lot of information as well as empathy and support.

Once the facts have been assimilated, the task of adjustment can begin. The parents need to see beyond the baby's problem to the little person beneath. The single malformation often throws the whole baby out of focus — for a few days the parents can only see the cleft palate. The process of grieving can slow down the acceptance of the baby and make the task of planning the future even harder.

Inevitably, the baby as a special and unique personality will emerge. The bonds form as strongly as ever, and the incredible resilience of human nature reveals itself.

LOSING A BABY

Words cannot describe the pain of the loss of a baby. A stillbirth is just as traumatic, the loss of a baby you have never met face to face, but whom you know intimately.

After the baby has gone, there are few memories to help validate his life and make it seem more real, so the following steps are important. Try, if possible, to get photographs of the baby, to hold his image for the future. Try to get some physical contact with your baby, even after death. Within every bereaved parent there is a 'cuddle that must come out' and it is important to hold him and to say goodbye, even if, at the time, this just seems to make it hurt more. Lastly, arrange a funeral, just like you would for any other member of the family. This too, underlines that the baby was a real person, loved and accepted by the family.

Remember, also, your poor friends. Some of them have no idea how to talk to you about your tragedy. They want to comfort you but they don't know how to start. They don't know whether to mention the baby or to avoid the subject altogether.

They may delay phoning you while they try to figure it out. Suddenly weeks have passed and they are ashamed it's been so long and it becomes even more difficult for them to call. It's hard but you may have to call them. Tell them about the baby and say that it's all right for them to talk to you about him — and not to mind if you cry when they do. They will be glad you have made it easier for them and they in turn will make it easier for you with their love and support. Other people, with the best will in the world, will say the wrong thing — but they are doing their best, so try to ignore their clumsiness.

It is important to hold him and to say goodbye, even if, at the time, this just seems to make it hurt more. This underlines that the baby was a real person, loved and accepted by the family.

▼▼▼

No-one emerges from this experience unchanged. For some, marital relationships end, broken by the stress, while for others their marriage becomes even stronger. But for everyone, life is changed. Many parents will say that the baby they lost has taught them more about life than those babies who remained. The poignancy of death taught them about passion, thoughtfulness and respect for life. As we regard birth with wonder and awe, mixed with joy and thankfulness, so death is on the other side of the coin, equally full of wonder and awe, but mixed with loss and finality.

It is the juxtaposition of these two staggering events that makes the loss of a newborn so difficult to assimilate.

The adjustment to the loss of a baby takes from several months to years and, unfortunately, it gets worse before it gets better. Most parents feel that they are coping far less well after a few weeks than they did immediately following the birth, as their body and mind gradually stop protecting them from feeling the full force of the loss. They may exhibit weird thoughts and behaviour, such as the desire to search for the baby or the need to protect the baby's grave from the weather. All these feelings are an adjustment and part of recovery.

It is a mistake to take drugs (including tranquillisers) to blunt the pain. When the drugs are stopped, the pain returns and while it remains denied it will affect other parts of life and relationships.

Eventually it has to be faced. When it is, the parents will experience intense mood swings. The so-called pangs of grief will plunge them into misery and sadness. These pangs usually continue to be painful but as the months go by they will occur less often. Though nothing can decrease the pain of loss, the best help is talking to each other or to someone who cares and understands. Loving relationships can be made or broken in such crises. As time passes, the parents usually find that they suffer pangs at different times and the depressed one doesn't wish to disturb the coping one with his or her sadness. Communication slows down and the couple can drift apart.

Do not protect your partner from your feelings. You are in this together. As time goes on, you will realise that the human mind has healing capacities far beyond anything you can imagine. The deep physical pain of your loss diminishes and the memory of your baby becomes a precious part of your past, remembered with love but without hurt — a soft ache which is the sad price some have to pay to try and achieve the joys of parenthood.

Then perhaps it is time to think of another pregnancy.

ZEN AND THE ART OF PARENTING

With children, as with our own life, every age has its special joys as well as those aspects we would prefer to forget. It is tempting to consider every stage our babies go through as merely preparation for the next phase of development.

Suddenly they look us in the eye and say goodbye — and we wonder where their childhood went. Their childhood happened while we were waiting for them not to do this or that, to be a bit more mature, and not get in our way so much. It happened when they screamed all night with earache, when they ran their tricycle into the furniture and when they refused to go to bed and stay there.

Our babies are our immortality, right here and now. They are also the best personal growth experience available. Anybody who wants to tread a spiritual pathway that will hold up a mirror to the person he or she truly is, need search no further than having a baby. There is no better teacher anywhere. We can be anyone we like to our friends — compassionate, patient, sensible — but our little ones will see through the facade and show us who we really are. Like no-one else, our babies can push our secret, psychic buttons.

Parenthood is an essential part of existence, for those who wish to grow and for those who would rather avoid it.

Don't miss the opportunity or the experience.

I wish you joy and enough sleep.

Glossary

Ammonia acrid smelling, skin irritating chemical produced by bacterial action (usually from the stool) acting on the urine.

Analgesic painkiller.

Carobel extract of carob bean, similar in effect to arrowroot, used for thickening milk.

Cartilage white elastic substance attached to joint-bone surfaces and other parts of the skeleton.

Cleft palate defect in formation of the palate, leaving a fissure in its surface.

Coagulation blood clotting.

Colostrum the first milk secreted by the breast, rich in antibodies and protein but poor in volume and calories.

Congenital present at and existing from the time of birth.

Conjunctivitis inflammation of membrane lining the eyelids and covering the eyeball.

Contraindication indication against a particular treatment.

Dextrostix or BM sticks bedside method of measuring sugar level in blood.

Distension swelling.

Down's Syndrome specific congenital disorder affecting all body tissues, caused by genetic accident.

Eczema reaction of skin with itching, redness and scaling.

Engorged excessively full.

Excision remove surgically.

Excoriation superficial loss of area of skin.

Fontanelle membrane-covered space at junction of bones of skull.

Gastroenteritis infection of the bowel, characterised by vomiting and/or diarrhoea, caused by bacteria or viruses.

Granulation soft, rounded mass of healing tissue.

Haemorrhage bleeding.

Heartburn pain caused by action of stomach acid on inflamed oesophagus.

Homeopathy system of alternative medicine that treats disease conditions by giving the body tiny quantities of substances that produce similar symptoms to those of the disease.

Hydrocortisone naturally-occurring hormone, one of whose effects is to reduce inflammation.

Lactose sugar of milk.

Leboyer French obstetrician who developed and publicised a mode of delivery that uses a quiet, dimly-lit environment to minimise psychological trauma to the baby.

Malformation defective formation of body tissues.

Maltogen a dried extract of malt sugars fortified with vitamin B1.

Maxolon or Bethanecol drugs which act on the valve mechanisms of the stomach and oesophagus.

Meconium dark green mucus-like material in the intestine of the fetus.

Mucus slimy secretion from the mucus membrane.

Neurological disorder disease state relating to the brain or nerves.

Nystatin or Mycostatin antibiotic that works against the fungus candida (thrush).

Ophthalmologist eye surgeon.

Oxytocin hormone secreted by the pituitary which stimulates contraction of the uterus.

Pertussis whooping cough.

Phototherapy treatment of jaundice that uses light to break down the bilirubin in the skin.

Pigmentation deposit of colouring matter within the skin.

Posset regurgitating the burp.

Projectile vomiting vomiting whereby stomach contents are thrown a distance.

Pustules small white pimples of infection.

Sun kicks outmoded and potentially dangerous exposure of the baby to the sun for short periods.

Saline solution of common salt in water with the same concentration as in body tissue. To make up: dissolve 2 level teaspoons of salt in 1 litre of water (1 level teaspoon in 1 pint of water).

Sorbolene a bland white emulsifying cream.

Spasm a sudden involuntary muscle contraction.

Spina bifida congenital defect of the spinal cord and/or spinal column at the lower end of the spine.

Tibia main leg bone below the knee.

Ultrasound medical imaging technique that uses sound waves instead of x-rays.

Urea end product of the body's protein metabolism.

INDEX